E. L. Edelstein

Anorexia Nervosa and Other Dyscontrol Syndromes

Springer-Verlag
Berlin Heidelberg New York
London Paris Tokyo

Professor Dr. E. L. Edelstein
20 Rav Berlin
Jerusalem 92503, Israel

ISBN-13:978-3-540-19281-7 e-ISBN-13:978-3-642-73700-8
DOI: 10.1007/978-3-642-73700-8

Library of Congress Cataloging-in-Publication Data. Edelstein, E. L. (Elieser Ludwig), 1922–
Anorexia nervosa and other dyscontrol syndromes / E. L. Edelstein. p. cm. Includes index.
ISBN-13:978-3-540-19281-7 (U.S.)
1. Anorexia nervosa. 2. Eating disorders. I. Title. [DNLM: 1. Appetite Disorders. WM 175 E21a]
RC552.A5E34 1988 616.85'2–dc19 DNLM/DLC 88-39903

2125/3130-543210

This book is dedicated to my teachers,
among them my patients,
to my sons, Amos, Ron and Arnon
and to my wife Lea.

The unusual opportunities and generous facilities provided
by the Institute for Advanced Study (Wissenschaftskolleg) Berlin
played a substantial role in the creation of this monograph.

Preface

> What is that which gleams through me and smites my heart without wounding it? I am both a-shudder and a-glow.
>
> St. Augustine

It is wonder and awe that I feel in view of the individual's power to create self-therapeutic devices. This book is the saga of these young individuals, who change and recreate the shape and dimensions of their bodies in a quest to achieve and finally demonstrate autonomy.

Ironically, it seems that they can go on living thanks to their excessive behavior, their hunger, and their deviances. They exhibit an extreme polarity, an "either-or": the thrill of excesses, the joy of giving in to pleasure, versus masochistic enjoyment and pride curbing, procrastinating and mastering these impulses almost to the absolute by simple force of effort and sublimatory strength. Somewhat alien to the medical profession, these maladies are self-induced, and only make sense if their symbolism is recognized and understood using a hermeneutic approach. It aptly reflects their interaction with other objects, both human and nonhuman.

The anorectic girl, to whom the book is specifically devoted, rejects any human bond in a masochistic way and also denies that her own body is a worthwhile object that deserves to be cared for. On the other hand, her body and its expressions are virtually under the most potent overcontrol. Thus, the narrative of the anorectics is strongly related to their incessant suffering, which is again of their own creation.

As a therapist, I attempt to describe and understand the essentially chaotic, but seemingly organized life history of anorectics in all its subtleties. I am grateful to all the patients who were tolerant enough to bear with my presence and "insatiable" curiosity while I was continuously trying to delve into the depths of their unconscious worlds. This is why I can tell their stories with more hope. I was able to feel and transmit hope in these long treatment processes because the anorectics provided me with new ideas, helping me to create hypotheses which gave me the renewed patience to go on and eventually be of some help. It is thus, in essence, the story of pain sustained by renouncing pleasure.

Jerusalem, October 1988 E. L. Edelstein

Contents

CHAPTER 1

Introduction

"There is no virtue in penance and fasting which waste the body; they are only fanatical and monkish."

Immanuel Kant, Lecture at Königsberg 1775

Anorexia nervosa is defined in the *DSM-III-R Diagnostic Criteria* as an eating disorder, or as a subclass of childhood and adolescent disorders. Besides the purely descriptive aspect, we believe that a wider conceptualization of this illness is in order. This belief stems from years of clinical work, research, and curiosity in the field of eating disorders in general and anorexia nervosa in particular. As a result of this intensive study, as well as of the research of others, we have arrived at the conclusion that anorexia nervosa belongs to a whole spectrum of hunger-driven illnesses. These illnesses all show elements of dyscontrol or ill-control of drives. The drives which are seen to be in need of control are such vitally essential ones as hunger, thirst, and sleep and such nonvital drives as sex and aggression, and their derivatives. The control devices used (as part of the ego function) include qualitatively and quantitatively different coping mechanisms such as undercontrol, overcontrol and dyscontrol (deviancy in control). Other behavioral disorders of this type include bulimia, obesity, drug abuse, activity addiction, and gambling.

Such issues can be compared and contrasted in the various manifestations of the dyscontrol syndrome. Anorexia is a model of overcontrol and a total supression of hunger. It incorporates fantasies of conversion into a neutral being, in which the body is used for masochistic purposes and the expression of self-hatred. In contrast, obesity is a model of loss of control. It is manifested by an ever-present feeling of hunger. Eating is used to express both love and aggression. Bulimia, which combines aspects of both anorexia and obesity, can be seen as a model of temporary loss of control within the context of compulsive overcontrol. Finally, drug addiction is a model of rebellion against self-control. The drug addict feels stimulus hunger and uses chemical compounds as magic devices, turning drugs into object equivalents, as drives turn into drive equivalents in the quest for drugs.

All the disturbances belonging to dyscontrol syndromes have real psychosomatic manifestations, in the most concrete sense of the word. The nutritional system is explicitly involved in communication with the external world. These disturbances are characterized by morbid cravings or hunger together with insatiability. This produces an intolerance of tension which can be overtly expressed by specific eating mannerisms or by decathecting from bodily needs.

Coping by compulsive rituals, self-destructive behavior, and omnipotent fantasies are frequent.

This book will be devoted primarily to looking at the causes and the effects of anorexia nervosa. However, since we believe that this disorder belongs to the wide spectrum of dyscontrol syndromes we shall, throughout the book, point out the similarities or differences that anorexia nervosa shares with obesity and drug abuse. This will be done through (a) a review of the historical significance of anorexia, showing that it is an ancient disease with its own idiosyncratic symptoms which result from various historical periods and social contexts, (b) looking at the biological and psychic processes which result from eating, and (c) examining the use of therapeutic practices and the attitudes of therapists in the treatment of anorexia.

Anorexia nervosa is a behavior disorder, manifesting itself mainly in eating and incorporating behavior as well as in the fear of becoming obese. It deals with impulses, excitement, stimulus barriers, control, and autonomy. Its implications are individual, social, and biological. In anorexia there may be a denial of some environmental and intrapsychic mechanisms, and a need to fill out the void created by this denial in which somatic processes of an infantile or even an archaic character take over.

Early learned mechanisms, namely eating, feeding, and incorporating, can express in symbolic ways feeling, volitional states, and wishes for autonomy and independence. These transformations naturally also touch on known biological mechanisms. The pure pathophysiology is not clear, in spite of the numerous facts relating to oscillating, temporary hypo-, or hyperfunctions in various systems. Consequently, because of the heterogeneity and the mixture of psychosomatic elements with personality regression, there is a great deal of controversy about the types of treatment recommended for patients suffering from anorexia and about their results.

We believe that the mind and body are holistically united. When some disintegrating event happens, the organism has to adapt on various levels, often by what we designate as early and regressive mechanisms. As a result, a certain disequilibrium of the former state may be produced between the psychic and the somatic part, or, in other words, a different role-taking by various psychic and/or somatic elements is produced.

The English designation is from the Greek term anorexia. In German it is called *Magersucht.* Any addiction is called *Sucht* in German. It is interesting to note that the term for anorexia is thinness-addiction (Magersucht), just like obesity *(Fettsucht)* or drug addiction *(Drogensucht).* The word *Sucht* stems from Middle High German, Old German, and Old Saxon *Suht, socht,* in Swedish *sot.* The German word *Siech* is like sick in English. One would assume that *Sucht* is connected with *suchen,* looking for something. From the term *Sucht,* meaning sickness, also stems the term *Seuche,* (a mostly epidemic) sickness (Kluge 1975).

Another interpretation of the term *Sucht* (Nils 1934) is that this group of words has to do with the German *Saugen,* which means to suck. He uses a citation that our forefathers believed that sickness was caused by sucking demons. *Sukana,* in Gothic *siukan,* actually meant to be sucked.

The earliest description of anorexia nervosa was ascribed to the Genovese physician *Simone Porta O. Portio* who lived around 1500 (Thomä 1967).

Richard Morton in 1689 in England published a paper about it, describing amenorrhea, lack of appetite, constipation, extreme emaciation and overactivity, a treatise of consumption.

Whitt, another eighteenth century English neurologist, published his book in 1767 and alluded obviously to anorexia nervosa.

Naudean, a French physician published a lengthy description of a fatal case in 1789.

E. Charles Lasegue, Professor of Clinical Medicine in Paris, published in 1873 *On hysterical anorexia (orexis* = desire, yearning*).*

W. Gull of London published his paper in 1874 on "apepsia hysterica."

Huchard in 1883 in France called the disease anorexia mentale.

Lasegue and Gull both thought that in some way also the family was responsible.

Pierre Janet in 1903 described a case of mental anorexia in his book *Les obsessions et la psychasthènique.* Psychasthenia is an obsessional form of disgust with one's own body. He found that the patient refused to play a feminine sex role. He was invited to Harvard Medical School in 1906–1907 for a series of 15 lectures. One of them was devoted to "hysterical anorexia." He felt that there was fundamentally a deep psychological disturbance.

André Thomä was the first to describe it as a syndrome in 1909. *Morris Simmonds* from Hamburg was the first who turned to an organic concept. He described a fatal case of anorexia (as he called it cachexia), in whom at autopsy he found a destructive or atrophic lesion of the anterior lobe of the pituitary. The female patient had been pregnant. Since then, for many years, it was called Simmond's cachexia.

E. Kylin in 1937 was probably the first who described systematically 50 cases of emaciation of girls in puberty. He still thought that it was a pituitary disease as had been assumed earlier.

Palmer (1972) called it *dietary chaos syndrome. Russell* (1979) used *bulimia nervosa. Crisp* (1979) employed *abnormal normal weight control. Van de Wiele* (1977) named it the *pubertal starvation-amenorrhoea.*

Women and Diseases: The Specific Feminine Aspect

Since the first description of anorexia nervosa, it has been considered to be a women's disease, either of pubertal girls or of pregnant women. It was described as nonacceptance of female sexuality. The earliest description of anorexia nervosa is ascribed to the Genovese physician Simone Porta O. Portio, who lived around 1500. Throughout the seventeenth and eighteenth centuries anorexia nervosa was recognized as a physical disorder with a physiologic basis. In 1903 Pierre Janet described a case of mental anorexia in his book *Les obsessions et la psychasthénique*. He described psychasthenia as an obsessional form of disgust with one's own body. He found that the patient refused to play a feminine sex role. Freud, in the beginning, called it "melancholia of the sexually immature."

Historically, women were always seen to be much more troubled by sexually linked diseases, especially by birth fever, infertility, dysmenorrhea, genital trouble, hysteria, migraine, and frigidity. Cancer was once considered mainly a women's disease. This was probably because the "external" recognizable cancer variations, such as breast cancer and bleeding diseases like cervical cancer, were more easily diagnosed. Similarly, during the mid-nineteenth century, tuberculosis was seen as the epitome of a women's disease. Often twice as many women died of it than men. For every 100 women aged 20 in 1865, more than five would be dead of tuberculosis by the age of 30.

This belief in women's susceptibility to disease was expressed in the nineteenth century ideal of the woman. Sickness was seen as feminine. The female consumptive did not lose her feminine identity: she embodied it – bright eyes, long lashes, translucent skin, and cherry-red lips. The female consumptive was romanticized. For the woman, being sick was on the one hand a flight from real life, while on the other hand it offered an erotization of the body as a whole, including spiritual elements of seduction.

These attitudes towards women were primarily the result of male fears and the acting out of those fears in society. Male fear of female sexual power and prowess is widespread. It seems that the mere existence of the uterus, its hidden productivity, and its "life of its own" pose a magical threat to men. Reproduction and sexuality seemed to stimulate men's fantasies and their resistance. Female sexuality has been seen as a curse; the very idea of a sexual woman was anxiety-provoking in the Middle Ages and in later periods. At the time of the Inquisition women by the thousands were declared witches, usually for being too independent or assertive. Competent women were seen as a threat to male omnipotence and mastery, and by a curious form of projection, active sexual women were accused of being evil. Sex itself was feared and abhorred when initiated by the woman. Pregnant women, birthing women, as well as menstruating women were thought of as poisonous and harmful. This can be seen especially in the practices of ancient and primitive societies.

In this context of beliefs the phenomenon of "churching" is particularly interesting. This is a religious practice by which a new mother is subject to various restrictions for 4–6 weeks after delivery in order to decontaminate her, with the aim of permitting reentry into society. This custom, which can be seen as a sort of exorcism, was found among the rites of the Christian church until the time of the Reformation, and was continued by the Anglican and Catholic churches until the beginning of the twentieth century. A form of this rite is continued by Orthodox Jews to this day. It is based on the passage in the Old Testament (Leviticus 12:2–8) which states that "A women shall be unclean for 7 days after birth of a boy and for 14 days after birth of a girl. For a further 33 days (when a boy) or for 66 days (in case of a girl) the mother shall not enter the sanctuary." After that period the woman was to make an offering, at which time she was to be considered once again "clean."

Canonic law makes it clear that a woman is not allowed to fill any high post within the church because of her menstruation and other bodily changes. It is intriguing to question the meaning and purpose of these various restrictions on pregnant, birthing, and menstruating women which are found in diverse cultures and religions. Can they be seen merely as attempts to maintain fertility and decrease the pleasurable aspects of sexual behavior? Or is the loss of blood, like the loss of semen, seen as an abomination since it is the loss of a precious life substance? Finally, can the restrictions be seen as a manifestation of the fear that men have of the openness of the female organ with its various discharges?

The Female Body: Social Aspects

Adolescence is an important phase in life, a period in which many changes take place, both in physical form and in abstract thinking and imagining. Adolescent girls seem to have many more subjective and objective difficulties than boys. As the young woman starts her monthly cycle she becomes, by that event, different in her biological and psychological functions from men. It is during adolescence that girls are subjected to the current standards of beauty, which demand a certain body image, an image which is based on male society and its wishes and values.

Women, as the so-called weaker sex, were controlled by male wishes. They had to be attractive at all times, according to the dictates of a specific society, culture, and epoch. These notions of feminine beauty have changed drastically. During the Renaissance voluptuous women were the ideal, whereas in Victorian times women had to be pale, fragile, and gracious. At the end of the nineteenth century, however, women were expected to be taller and rather athletic.

In the beginning of this century, the boy-like, graceful ideal predominated, as epitomized by Mary Pickford. In the 1920s, the flat-breasted, thin woman was in fashion. From the 1930s to the 1960s, the sexy type was again idealized; "sexy" meaning having big, round breasts, a narrow waist, and long legs. At the same time women were expected to grow thinner and thinner. This trend may have had something to do with the advent of easy-to-use birth control and the redefinition of women more as sex symbols than as mothers. Birth control also gave women autonomous control over their bodies and pregnancy, and thereby mastery over frequent changes in form.

In our own era, women's bodies, or even parts of their bodies, have been used for selling products. The female bust, hips, and seductive looks under painted eyelids have all been connected with advertisements for the sale of cars, alcohol, cigarettes, etc. Like a fetishist society, parts of the female body are being separated and used for propaganda (Orbach 1982).

Besides fulfilling a sexual role, women are also expected to be the preparers and providers of food. No matter how a woman strives for independence this role is, by definition, feminine.

By adolescence, girls feel the beginnings of societal pressure to conform to the role-model of the attractive woman and nurturer. As is natural during adolescence, there is a need to rebel and to become autonomous and independent. But rebellion, autonomy, and independence are not accepted female characteristics. Nevertheless, some women do rebel, sometimes by choosing to reject society's feminine ideal. This is done by deciding to control and master every drive, especially the most basic drives – hunger and sexuality. There may be an element of desiring to be like a Spartan, the ideal man whose strength lies in not yielding, and not yielding to the most essential and vital drives means that one is really omnipotent.

Hunger and sexuality are seen by the anorectic as a form of dependency. It is through rebelling against these drives that the anorectic is able to show her strength. Habermass (1986) believes that the anorectic ideal of the thin body is an extreme form of the present beauty type, and that in not eating the rejection of dependence is reflected.

The need to reject dependence applies to all addictions, behavioral excesses, or insatiability. The model of dependency – its first instance and imprinted memory – is infantile hunger; the infant demands immediate satisfaction. Infantile hunger and its satisfaction relate to pure impulse, and the infant is unable to tolerate disappointment or delay.

The various manifestations of addictive addictions result in various personality disorders. The anorectic practices the utmost control over wild impulses and their possible breakthrough. In order not to lose control and eat, they even turn on a delusional system, in order to prove that the body really does not need any addition of food. The bulimic suffers from a similar disturbance which is manifested in a different way. Bulimics give in to the inevitability of the drive and its satisfaction. The food is erotized and turned into an object, just as with the anorectic, but the bulimic practices a temporary game of loss of control and therefore satisfies the hunger drive, with all its oral and genital implications. The drug-abusing youngster is somewhat further away from these fundamental axes. The drug is used instead of the real incorporated object, the food. The drug is erotized and the user seduces it or feels seduced by it. Drug addicts cannot tolerate tension or suffer psychic pain. Drugs are related to as living objects, with the user getting caught up in a vicious circle of need, losing the element of control altogether.

Physical Diagnosis

The physical diagnosis of anorexia nervosa can be based on the following:

1. The illness begins between the ages of 10 and 30 years, usually before age 25.
2. A loss of at least 25% of body weight (original body weight) and a body weight 15% below normal for age and height (as obtained from Metropolitan Life Insurance Policy Scales for normal weight) are seen.
3. A distorted attitude and behavior towards eating, food, and weight is displayed and remains in spite of hunger, warnings, threats, etc. This distorted attitude and behavior manifests itself in:
   - Denial of illness and failure to recognize nutritional needs
   - Apparent enjoyment in losing weight
   - A desired body image of extreme thinness
   - Unusual hoarding or handling of food
4. At least two of the following symptoms are seen:
   - Amenorrhea of at least 3 months' duration
   - Lanugo hair
   - Bradycardia (at least 60/min resting pulse)
   - Hypothermia
   - Episodes of bulimia
   - Vomiting, possibly self-induced
   - Periods of overactivity
   - Acrocyanosis
5. There is compulsive self-administration of laxatives or diuretics.
6. No other major psychiatric disorder, such as a major affective disorder or schizophrenia, is present.
7. The subject has no known medical illness that could account for the anorexia and the weight loss:
   - *Cardiovascular*
     Bradycardia
     Hypotension
     Arrhythmia
   - *Gastrointestinal*
     Decreased gastric emptying
     Constipation
     Elevated hepatic enzymes
   - *Hematologic*
     Anemia

Leukopenia
Thrombocytopenia
- *Renal*
  Increased blood urea nitrogen
  Decreased glomerular filtration rate
  Renal calculi
  Edema
- *Endocrine/metabolic*
  Amenorrhea
  Osteoporosis
  Euthyroid sick syndrome
  Decreased norepinephrine secretion
  Decreased somatomedin C
  Elevated growth hormone
  Decreased or erratic vasopressin secretion
  Abnormal temperature regulation
  Hypercarotenemia
- *Physical Examination*
  Skeletal muscle atrophy
  Active in spite of emaciation
  Changing axillar and pubic hair – lanugo hair
  Arterial hypotension
  Bradycardia
  Constipation
  Dental caries
  Facial edema – sudden reversal with normal eating
  Hands and feet bluish
  Nails brittle
  Subcutaneous edema is rare
  (unlike in other forms of malnutrition)
  In a later stage feet edematous
- *Laboratory Tests*
  Light anemia
  Blood sugar low in 50% of patients
  Insulin tolerance often abnormal
  Liver and renal functions normal
  Oliguria
  Sella turcica normal
- *Endocrine*
  Amenorrhea and drop in basal metabolic rate
  Lower than normal 17-ketosteroids and 11-oxysteroids
  Radioactive iodine tests: normal thyroid function
  and normal protein-bound iodine level

Normal response to ACTH-stimulation
(Amenorrhea is due to isolated gonadotropic insufficiency due to a purely psychogenic mechanism involving the corticothalamohypophyseal system or due to a general physical depression. Amenorrhea is accompanied by a reduced elimination of estrogen. The ovaries shrink, the endometrium becomes fibrotic, and the vaginal mucosa atrophies.)

– *Electrolytes*
As adipose tissue shrinks, the percentage of water in the body as a whole increases. At the same time the total amount of potassium (mainly intercellular) tends to decrease as a result of muscular atrophy, while the total amount of sodium tends to increase. When purgatives are being taken and vomiting exists, there will be hypokalemia and hyponatremia, causing dehydration and finally metabolic alkalosis. The azotemia is prerenal.
Carotenemic skin is a common clinical finding. However, in other forms of organic weight loss low levels of carotene and vitamin A have been found. So, in anorexia there may be either an increase in dietary carotene and vitamin A intake or an acquired defect in the metabolism of vitamin A (Feighner et al. 1972).

General Characteristics

Anorectic women seem to be characteristically unconcerned about their deviant physical condition. Their behavior may seem withdrawn, strange, critical, and intolerant of the criticism of others. Their thin, emaciated bodies look skeleton-like, with protruding bones. The facial muscles are tight, as there is no subcutaneous fat to cushion them. The legs have no form and are like matchsticks. The breasts disappear and the obdomen appears concave. Head and lanugo hair may fall out. With slight changes in temperature acrocyanosis will appear. Anorectic girls and women are usually of average or higher intelligence, with typical coping mechanisms: denial, repression, isolation, and compulsive ritualism. Memory and the ability to concentrate are present; thinking is rational and fast. Emotions are avoided as much as possible. Masochistic tendencies are prevalent.

Anorectics are active, which so contrasts with expectations from such weak bodies that they seem to be hyperactive. They are usually excellent employees, becoming absorbed and addicted to their work.

Studies have found that anorectics express delusional body images, denying their deviance and believing that they look normal or even fat (Bruch 1973). They may also fail to recognize certain sensory stimuli. This may be the result of the exclusive need to control, which overpowers any other wish or anxiety. Anorectics express a fear, almost phobic in character, of impulses and sensory stimulation, including sexual stimulation. One can hardly speak about a prodroma of the disease, especially since the majority of anorectics deny the disease's existence and therefore refuse to see a physician.

The first apparent symptom is the overt or covert refusal of food. This may be done by eating extremely slowly or by refusing to eat with other members of the family. Anorexia is also characterized by a strong desire to lose weight through vomiting or through the self-administration of laxatives or diuretics. The anorectic will sometimes avoid food altogether, while at the same time providing food for others. Anorectics are known to hoard food, especially when hospitalized and treated by inexperienced therapists (Crisp 1979). The family situation may be controlled by the anorectic member using games and obsessive-compulsive rituals. This is done in order to break the family's resistance to the anorectic's behavior.

It was generally believed that anorectics stemmed mostly from the upper middle class of Western society. Recently, however, cases of anorexia are being reported from non-Western countries and among classes other than the middle class (Buchan and Gregory 1984; Thomas and Szmukler 1985).

The overall impression of physicians and psychologists working in the field is that in the last few years the number of patients suffering from anorexia nervosa has increased significantly (Health and Public Policy Committee 1986). In spite of this dramatic increase, however, physicians exhibit very complex, contradictory attitudes towards anorexia. Vanderdeycken and Vanderlinden (1983) believe that most physicians do not consider anorectics as having a genuine illness and see them as impostors, although they know the danger to life that advanced anorexia can cause. On the other hand, this state originates from consciously and wilfully induced starvation so that doctors are subject to doubts about treatment motivation. This confusion is aggravated by the fact that most anorectics usually do not seek treatment of their own free will, and openly declare that they have no interest in cooperating in their own treatment.

References

Bruch H (1973) Eating disorder: obesity, anorexia nervosa and the person within. Basic, New York

Buchan T, Gregory LD (1984) Anorexia nervosa in a black Zimbabwean. Br J Psychiatry 145:326–330

Crisp AH (1979) Abnormal normal weight control: fatness, metabolism and sexual behavior. In: Carenza L, Zichella L (eds) Emotion and reproduction, 20a. Academic, London, pp 215–237

Feighner JP, Robins E, Guze SB, Woodruff RA, Winokur J, Munoz R (1972) Diagnostic criteria for use in psychiatric research. Arch Gen Psychiatry 27:57

Freud S (1932) New introductory lectures. Lecture 33. Hogarth Press, London

Habermass T (1986) Zur Bedeutung der Schlankheit im Erleben Magersüchtiger. Psychother Med Psychol 36:69–74

Health and Public Policy Committee, American College of Physicians (1986) Position paper: eating disorders: anorexia nervosa and bulimia. Ann Intern Med 105:790–794

Janet P (1903) Les obsessions et la psychasthenique. Alcan, Paris

Kluge F (1975) Etymologisches Wörterbuch der deutschen Sprache, 21 edn. de Gruyter, Berlin

Nils L (1934) Norsk tidskr. Sprogvidensk 7:170

Orbach S (1987) Hungerstreik. ECON, Düsseldorf

Palmer RL (1972) Dietary chaos syndrome: a useful new term? Br J Med Psychol 52:57–63

Russell G (1979) Bulimia nervosa: an ominous variant of anorexia nervosa. Psychol Med 9:429–448

Shorter E (1982) A history of women's bodies. Basic, New York, p 242

Thomä H (1967) Anorexia nervosa. International University Press, New York

Thomas JP, Szmukler GI (1985) Anorexia nervosa in patients of Afro-Caribbean extraction. Br J Psychiatry 146:653–656

Vanderdeycken W, Vanderlinden J (1983) Denial of illness and the use of self-reporting measures in anorexia nervosa patients. Int J Eating Disorders 2(4):101–107

Van de Wiele RL (1977) Anorexia nervosa and the hypothalamus. Hosp Pract 12:45–51

CHAPTER 2

Fasting – Asceticism

> "There is nothing the body suffers that the soul may not profit by!"
>
> George Meredith 1828–1909: Diana of the Crossways

The phenomenon of the fasting anorectic is the result of various societal, psychologic, and physical factors. These include society's pressure on women to be thin, and the disgust many women feel towards their own bodies. Fasting also improves mood, causing euphoria and often the feeling of being in control. It is frequently the fear of being out of control, of being unable to stop eating, that initiates a period of fasting. In turn, the ability to control this most vital drive, eating, is seen as proof of the ability to control less vital drives such as sex. Fasting is also used by adolescent girls as a way to control the bodily changes which signal the onset of adulthood and is therefore used to deny their feminine identity.

Fasting

For human beings, the act of fasting is usually the result of either physical conditions beyond individual control (i.e., famine), or societal conditions such as religious practices. As we have mentioned, fasting is a part of many religious sects, though it is usually limited to specific days, and is used for the purpose of metaphorically and spiritually cleansing the body and soul. The conscious decision of the individual to fast is quite rare and is usually the result of certain motivational states, such as the need to unconsciously hurt or destroy oneself, or to gain control and power over essential drives and to be able to inhibit these drives at will.

The physiological changes induced by fasting include a sudden transition to a different state of maintenance and the resulting change in the level of adaptation. In the initial stage of hyperfunction the system will adapt to the new phase. A stress reaction follows, which causes a rise in cortisol and catecholamine levels. This is followed by a transitional stage from short-span adaptation to long-term adaptation, which is a correlate of reduced stress. Finally, a new adaptation level is reached, with the normalization of cortisol and catecholamine levels.

A malignant stage is reached, however, when fasting is continued to the point of starvation, i.e., when all the body's reserves are used up. This results in functional insufficiency and damage to bodily organs by the depletion of adaptive forces.

Certain biochemical mechanisms start to work in the adaptation phase of fasting. Teleologically, it seems that one of the "aims" of the fasting body is to save glucose for the central nervous system (CNS). A reduction of proteolysis and the creation of ATP from fatty acids and keto-bodies also takes place. Jungermann and Mohler (1984) showed that in acute hunger states – within a short adaptation span – the CNS needs 144 g glucose, while when fasting it needs only 44 g glucose. Since the CNS can adapt to smaller amounts of glucose there is also consequently a saving of protein. Under conditions of acute hunger the liver produces 90% of the newly built glucose. But when fasting (long adaptation) is induced the liver produces only 60% of the newly built glucose, the rest coming from the kidneys. This is caused by the presence of keto-acidosis, a result of fasting. In this process of gluconeogenesis, ammonium is liberated from amino acids and is used for the neutralization of the urine.

Physiologic and Behavioral Adaptation

The question of whether there are any physiologic differences in the adaptation of the organism to enforced as opposed to voluntary fasting has been researched extensively. One of the earliest studies was conducted by Keys et al. (1950) on the behavior and emotional states of 36 volunteers in a condition of semi-starvation (defined as being half the required caloric intake). After only a few days, the subjects exhibited poor concentration, moodiness, depression, loss of ambition, and a general emotional instability. Some of the subjects displayed a combination of irritability and apathy. Often bizarre behavior resulted, such as compulsive feeding rituals and increased preoccupation with food. Finally, the feeling of hunger completely disappeared. This is in contrast to the mood of anorectics, who often display emotional states of euphoria, assertiveness, and hyperactivity, with an enhanced ability for abstract thinking.

In both starvation and anorexia nervosa, acute gastric dilatation was found by Dubois et al. (1984). Gastric fractional emptying rate and acid output were halved compared with healthy subjects. It was also found that acute cholinergic stimulation temporarily increased gastric acid output and fractional emptying rate in anorectics suggesting that the gastric smooth muscle and parietal cells remain responsive to cholinergic stimulation. However Dubois believes that the stimulated gastric parameters are less in anorexia nervosa, and that gastric effector cells may be atrophied or that the sensitivity of their cholinergic receptors decreased. Dubois, therefore, suggests cholinergic therapy as an adjuvant. Holzl and Lautenbacher (1984) used a more sophisticated and less penetrative method of measuring feeding response, by means of a variant of surface gastrography which avoided the adverse effects of intragastric pressure probes. They also found retarded gastric emptying in anorectics, which did not exist in dieting or fasting volunteers.

Several studies have tried to ascertain the possible influence of fasting on the body's immunological competence. In a WHO study (Scrimshaw et al. 1968) it was found that there seems to be a higher incidence of infectious diseases in malnutritional states. Suskind (1977) found that identifying this cause-effect relationship was not clear-cut, since environmental factors such as overcrowding, poor hygiene, and high psychosocial stress may increase susceptibility. In contrast Kjosen et al. (1975), using immunological techniques, found that infections are uncommon and viral diseases rare among anorectics. This seemed to be the result of a decrease in granulocyte response (Palmblad 1976), glucose oxidation, and bactericidal capacity. Gotch et al. (1975) and Palmblad et al. (1979) found some "granulocyte killing defect" in anorexia nervosa. Kjelberg et al. (1977) exposed volunteers of normal weight to 10 days of total energy deprivation. This resulted in a depression in serum levels of several acute-phase reactants – complement factor C3, haptoglobin, orosomucoid and transferrin – and a decrease of iron plasma levels. There was a depression of the DNA synthesis of blood lymphocytes and a decline in the bactericidal capacity and the alkaline phosphatase activity of blood neutrophils. On the other hand, there was no influence on the serum levels of IgM, IgA, IgE, C4, and haptoglobin, on the interferon-producing capacity and the subpopulation of blood lymphocytes, on the iron saturation index of serum transferrin, or on the skin's delayed hypersensitivity to purified protein derivative (PPD) and mumps antigen. Kim and Michael (1975) and Palmblad et al. (1979), being especially interested in anorectic patients and their fasting state, described changes in the serum complement system, mainly depressions of factors C1, C2, C3, C1 inactivator, the total hemolytic complement. C4 was found to be normal. In addition, plasma levels of complement factors 3 and 4 and orosomucoid and opsonic functions in anorexia nervosa were different from normal levels.

Another interesting study comparing normal fasting patients and anorectics was carried out by Fichter and Pirke (1984). The pituitary-hypothalamic function was tested in normal volunteers before and after a period of starvation and once again after their return to normal weight. Disturbances in endocrine function were detected in the hypothalamic-pituitary-adrenal axis, the luteinizing hormone (LH) secretory pattern, the thyroid-stimulating hormone (TSH) response to stimulation with thyrotropin-releasing hormone (TRH), basal growth hormone secretion, growth hormone response following stimulation with clonidine, and basal prolactin secretion. Their results supported the hypothesis that the endocrine disturbances reported in anorexia nervosa are not primary, but a consequence of reduced food intake or loss of body weight.

From these and numerous other studies it becomes clear that a significant period of fasting (10 days) causes an elevation of the levels of serum growth hormone, cortisol concentration, and urine output of epinephrine and norepinephrine. The serum thyroid hormone level falls. This seems to indicate that undereating will decrease previously normal host resistance. However, there seem to be different results to fasting by healthy and by sick people. For instance, Uden et al. (1980) found that total fasting for 7 days by patients with rheumatoid arthritis caused a rise of granulocyte function and increased bactericidal capacity.

Thus, the clinical significance of the reduced host defense variables is not quite clear. There have been claims that anorectics are less vulnerable to infectious disease. A similar "myth" existed concerning schizophrenics. This was usually the result of the fact that psychotics have little object relations with their surroundings and live to a great extent in an autistic world of their own. They are less interested in external influences, including those concerning their own bodies. In contrast, anorectics practice a Spartan-like behavior which includes strongly masochistic aspects and obstinacy in mastering their own needs. In addition, anorectics exhibit a high tolerance to sensory experiences such as pain, temperature, and hunger. Considering these behavioral manifestations, it is not surprising that anorectics are able to tolerate and ignore symptoms of illness.

In conclusion, the greater risk of infection or other physical trauma for anorectics is still a disputed subject and the results of the various studies cited above are equivocal. However, the psychosomatic aspect of probable differing immunological responses to different motivations for fasting can be substantiated.

Psychiatric Views on Asceticism

One of the primary psychiatric mechanisms of asceticism is behavior that can be termed "moral masochism." This can be seen as a behavioral norm, in contradistinction to the sexual perversion of masochism. The defense mechanisms involved in moral masochism are primarily denial and libidinization of suffering. The moral masochist does not want to suffer or to punish himself; nevertheless, he not only accepts, but even seeks suffering in order to achieve a feeling of narcissistic gratification and increased love-worthiness.

Freud states that there is no single satisfactory explanation for masochism. The principle of the renunciation of pleasure may be the aim of being loved for the suffering. Physical suffering can result in the achievement of a better sense of self-representation, i.e., in pain one feels one's existence. In contrast, moral masochism is a caricature of the Protestant ethic, which stresses discipline, hard work, and the denouncement of pleasure. The ego ideal, quite removed from the sensed ego, is an ideal of sacrifice, self-control, and victory over "lower" impulses. The danger is that asceticism can deviate from its acknowledged spiritual goal and degenerate into the obtaining of masochistic satisfaction from renunciation and self-mortification.

Examples from physiological or pathological conditions show the complex elements of stimulus and reaction which cause a combination of pain and pleasure. This can most easily be seen in dermatological lesions which itch. Itching is a subliminal, below-threshold pain. It is due to skin lesions, often caused by emotional responses such as tension, anxiety, and depression. No one needs to be convinced of the pleasure in scratching an itchy spot, often with an almost orgiastic satisfaction. Scratching is usually continued to the point of pain or over-irritation, and even this resulting pain seems to cause a pleasurable response.

Elements of sensuous pleasure mixed with anxiety and psychic pain have been observed and pointed out by many authors (e.g., Balint 1957). The Marquis de Sade, both in his own writings and in stories written about him by others, showed not only the perverse elements of sadism and masochism, but also the adventure of lust and pain. The ascetic self-torture in the Middle Ages, while formally considered as being hostile to the body and a victimization of the body for the soul, also contained an element of stimulatory excitement which would therefore negate the formal attitude of killing the body. Even in hypnosis, the pleasure of painful procedures can be induced when specific motivations, like guilt feelings, are evoked.

Self-discipline in adolescence is adaptive, but can increase to become extreme behavior. As Anna Freud states (Freud 1966): "the asceticism of puberty must be interpreted not as a series of repressive activities, qualitatively conditioned, but simply as a manifestation of the innate hostility between the ego and the instincts, which is indiscriminate, primary and primitive". Blos (1962) agrees with Freud and Fenichel that asceticism, with its origins in the Oedipal conflict, is a condition of adolescence. But he also adds to the theory the dimension of cultural influences and sees asceticism as more typical of European youth. In his study of the concept of chastity, Stern (1966) concurs with Blos's findings that ascetic practices are influenced by the cultural environment. Stern stated that although virginity has always been an ascetic ideal, it has been so for different reasons, which vary with changing religio-philosophical concepts. Gilberg (1974) sees the religious ascetic as saying: "If I can have mother (mother church), I will renounce much of the genital aspects of my sexuality."

Regression is the primary response of the ascetic's ego by the detachment from the material world through the renunciation of sensual satisfaction in general and of genital sexuality in particular. It is a returning of the ego-functioning to an earlier level of development. The blocking of genital outlet in asceticism tends to reactivate oral and anal levels of functioning. The pregenital phase is in fact bisexual, with the individual wishing for both male and female genital features. Together with the pregenital phase there are also the feelings of omnipotence and omniscience, as well as that of "omniactivity," since most ascetics experience a belief in the possession of great knowledge and the experience of absolute truth.

Asceticism can therefore be seen as the result of three psychological needs: (a) a defense against drive, (b) a defense against a sense of powerlessness, and (c) an expression of a wish for aesthetic and moral transcendence. This demarcation reinforces our notion of understanding the anorectic as one who exhibits an all-or-none attitude towards differentiated sex.

In relation to fasting and the tendency for asceticism in anorectic women, we shall review historical and religious attitudes towards fasting.

Religious Attitudes Toward Fasting

Judaism

Although the origins of the fasting practices of the Bible are obscure there are several theories which attempt to explain their purpose (see the Encyclopaedia Judaica 1972). Smith (1969) believes that fasting originated as a spiritual preparation for the partaking of a sacred meal. Tylor (1960) believes that fasting was used as a method for inducing a state of susceptibility to visions. And Gaster (1955) suggests that fasting was used as a means of providing new vitality during periods of human or nature's infertility.

Whatever its original origins and purpose, fasting by the Second Temple period (1st century A.D.) had become a part of religious practice with set guidelines and limitations. A philosophy of fasting existed wherein a fast without sincere repentance was seen as valueless and senseless. Fasting was also seen as an ascetic exercise, serving to purify man and bring him close to God. This conception of fasting closely resembled the concept of complete abstinence and asceticism, whose purpose was to induce ecstasy and apocalyptic visions and is found not only in the apocalyptic literature of the Second Temple period but also among certain circles of Talmudic rabbis, especially after the destruction of the Temple. This philosophy led to an exaggerated propagation of fasting, which in turn aroused a sharp reaction in general rabbinical literature. The rabbis condemned ascetic women, especially widows and young girls.

In Judaism, fasts were classified into three categories: (a) fasts decreed in the bible or instituted to commemorate biblical events, (b) fasts decreed by the rabbis, and (c) private fasts. Private fasts were also categorized: (a) on the anniversary of a parent's or teacher's death, (b) by the bride and groom on their wedding day, or (c) to avert the evil consequences of nightmares. The latter was the result of the belief in Talmudic times that bad dreams could have pernicious effects. This fast was regarded as necessitating such urgency that the rabbis permitted it even on the Sabbath. However, in later centuries the obligatory nature of this fast was mitigated by Halachic authorities.

Asceticism, the rigorous abstention from any form of self-indulgence, is based on the belief that renunciation of the desires of the flesh and self-mortification can bring man to a higher spiritual state. Asceticism never occupied an important place in the Jewish religion. Judaism did not believe that the freedom of man could be achieved only by the subjugation of the flesh, a belief which was central in religions based upon anthropological dualism. The only ascetic practice that Judaism does sanction, to a limited degree, is fasting. Fasting is to be used as an expression of remorse or sadness or as an act to aid concentration in prayer. The prophets emphasize over and over again the fact that fasting and the mortification of the body by themselves do not please God. The rabbis went even further: They consider asceticism and privation as a sin against the will of God; people should enjoy the gift of life.

Christianity

In the strictly orthodox Christian system, asceticism, while favoring austerity, does not disown the body but seeks its sanctification by its subjection to God's will. Christian philosophy struggled to maintain a monism in which the material world, no less than the spiritual, is God's creation. Evil is seen as the deprivation of good. The major heresies which influenced early Christianity sprang from mainly non-Christian, Eastern traditions, which viewed the phenomenal world as evil or illusory. The Gnostic, Arian, Manichaean, Priscillian, and Albigensian heresies all involved dualistic beliefs, and many practiced a type of asceticism which showed contempt for the body and the material world (Meddlicott 1969). As a result, the early Christians retreated behind their creed, felt infallible, associated the world with evil, retreated from pleasure, and prophesied doom. It is interesting to note that Christian theologians saw the lack of emphasis on asceticism in Judaism as proof of its inferior religious quality (Boussett 1966).

Buddhism

Buddhists make a conscious effort to retreat from the physical world in order to achieve Nirvana, the state of bodiless existence. Buddhism institutionalized asceticism and developed four ascetic steps in order to achieve a systematic suppression of all emotional life: self-induced melancholia, narcissism, apathy, and finally mental emptiness and uniformity. This final state is equivalent to Nirvana, the womblike state where one finds "no perception, no wishes, the peace, in which there is no death nor being reborn, no here, no beyond, only an intermediate kingdom that is even the end of sorrow" (Alexander 1931). Alexander suggested that Buddha's method of achieving the ascetic ideal was similar to psychoanalysis, but with a fundamental difference – Buddha denied reality.

Studies of religious fasts have proposed various explanations for its use in all major religions. Blumensohn (1933) proposed that fasting is a means of putting the individual into a personal relationship with the supernatural. Westermerck (1907), who made an extended study of fasting, proposed that fasting connected with mourning was the result of the fear of swallowing food polluted with the contagion of death. Westermerck also saw the intentional inducement of hunger as a way of returning to the parent-child relationship in the infantile situation. Thus, the hungrier the child (supplicant), the sooner the parent (God) would come. Dundes (1963) suggested that the use of fasting in marriage rituals was a result of the connection between hunger and love, i.e., the hungrier one is, the more love is needed and wanted.

Fasting Among Anorectics

Anorectics use fasting for two main purposes: (1) Fasting is a regression to the infantile connection with hunger and the demand for food, equaling love. It is a call for love from the parent (or God) by including hunger. It is also a way of remaining in the infantile state by refusing to grow up physically. (2) Fasting is a suppression of the pleasure of the flesh, with the idea that by suppressing hunger which is the most vital drive, other less vital drives, such as sex, can also be suppressed. This control of bodily drives is seen as a way of becoming clean or holy. There may also be a third use of fasting, namely, a rebellion against tradition, society and culture, and an identification with ascetic saints.

Women's use of their bodies to express the need for love, control, or rebellion can be seen as a result of historical and societal concepts of women and their bodies (Westermerck 1922). Women's bodies have been regarded as essentially sinful, defiled, and defiling. Women were seen as being filled with licentious sexual desire, seducing and corrupting men. According to Baker-Miller (1978), woman's social and psychological territory is essentially that of man's unresolved problems. Issues with which the dominant culture has never come to terms, e.g., sexuality, death, and the expression of emotion are handed over to the domain of women. Thus man is able to exorcize a demon of his own by punishing woman for her sexuality.

It is interesting to note the similarities in the motivations for anorectic behavior among religious women of the past and secular women of today. R.M. Bell (1985) in his book *Holy Anorexia* describes the lives of 261 holy women officially recognized by the Roman Catholic Church as saints, blesseds, venerables, or servants of God, from the period 1200 A.D. until the present. Of these 261 women, almost 100 displayed clear signs of anorexia. This is a description of the disease over 400 years old. The book is particularly useful for indicating the close similarity of anorexia symptoms, with due synchronicity to different social, cultural and religious attitudes.

Bell points out that in order to be holy in the Middle Ages it was necessary to have no needs, be they sexual, narcissistic, or nutritional. For women, the *sine qua non* for holiness was purity, which meant that all desires, including the desire for food, had to be obsessively avoided. This is a clear indication of the connection between holiness and starvation. Of the 42 Italian women from the thirteenth century who are recognized as saints, nearly half exhibited anorectic behavior patterns, as illustrated in the description of the lives of Angela of Foliguo, Margaret of Cortona and Veronica Giuliani (Orsola). These women felt driven to destroy their bodies, since they believed that if the flesh cannot be tamed it must therefore be obliterated. Since virgins and pious widows did not engage in sexual intercourse, food was the only thing that entered their bodies, and usually only when they were pressed to accede to the orders of their confessors.

In the epilogue of the book, William N. Davis tries to relate "holy anorexia" to present day anorexia (Bell 1985). Though in the accounts described there is no expressed striving for thinness or fear of fatness, the drive for holiness (spiritual perfection) exhibits the same hyperactivity and perfectionism that results from the present-day drive for bodily perfection. Davis stresses in particular the lack of understanding we have for female psychologic needs, and the use of the body as a form of rebellion against male dominance, both in the past and the present.

Asceticism in women can therefore be seen as an attempt to attain spirituality, goodness, or moral strength by punishing that part of themselves which women have been taught to see as both weak and sinful – the body. As Marilyn Lawrence (1979) put it: "Women's feelings are related to the position in which society faces them and to the taboos and denigrating explanations, with which it surrounds them. The self-disgust which a woman learns for her normal bodily processes, such as pregnancy and menstruation, the "choice" of labels to describe her sexuality (e.g. 'whore' or 'virgin', 'tight' or 'loose'); it is not difficult to understand why women associate their bodies with defilement and badness."

References

Alexander F (1931) Buddhistic training as an artificial catafonie. Psychoanal Rev 18:129–149
Baker-Miller J (1978) Toward a new psychology of women. Penguin, London
Balint M (1957) The doctor, the patient, and the illness. International Universities Press, New York
Bell RM (1985) Holy anorexia. The University of Chicago Press, Chicago
Blos P (1962) On adolescence: a psychoanalytic interpretation. Free, Glenco IL

Blumensohn J (1933) The fast among North American Indians. Am Anthropol 35:451–468
Bousset W (1966) In: Gressmann H (ed) Die Religion des Judentums in späthellenistischem Zeitalter. Mohr, Tübingen, pp 428–429
Brumberg JJ (1982) Chlorotic girls: a historical perspective on female adolescence. Child Dev 53:1468–1477
Dubois A, Gross HA, Ebert MH (1984) Gastric function in primary anorexia nervosa. In: Pirke KM, Ploog D (eds) The psychology of anorexia nervosa. Springer, Berlin Heidelberg New York
Dundes A (1963) Summoning deity through ritual fasting. The American Imago 20(3):213–220
Encyclopaedia Judaica, vol 6 (1972) Keter, Jerusalem, pp 676–683; 1190–1196
Fichter MM, Pirke KM (1984) Hypothalamic-pituitary function in starving healthy subjects. In: Pirke KM, Ploog D (eds) The psychology of anorexia nervosa. Springer, Berlin Heidelberg New York, pp 124–135
Freud A (1966) The ego and the mechanisms of defence. The writings of Anna Freud, vol 2. International Universities Press, New York
Gaster TH (1955) Festivals of the Jewish year, Sloane, New York, pp 190–211
Gilberg AL (1974) Asceticism and the analysis of a nun. J Am Psychoanal Assoc 22(2):381–393
Gotch FM, Spry CJF, Mowat A, Beeson PB, MacLennani CM (1975) Reversible granulocyte killing defect in anorexia nervosa. Clin Exp Immunol 21:244–249
Holzl R, Lautenbacher S (1984) Psychophysiological indices of the feeding response in anorexia nervosa patients. In: Pirke KM, Ploog D (eds) The psychobiology of anorexia nervosa. Springer, Berlin Heidelberg New York
Jungermann K, Mohler H (1984) Biochemie. Springer, Berlin Heidelberg New York, pp 233–298
Keys A, Brozek J, Henschel A, Michelson L, Taylor HL (1950) The biology of human starvation. University of Minneapolis Press, Minneapolis, pp 819–918
Kim Y, Michael AE (1975) Hypocomplementemia in anorexia nervosa. J Pediatr 87:582–585
Kjelberg J, Levy L, Palmblad J, Paulsson I, Theorell T, Yensen R (1977) Energy deprivation in man – methodological problems and possibilities. Acta Med Scand 201:9–13
Kjosen B, Bassoe HH, Myking O (1975) The glucose oxidation in isolated leucocytes from female patients suffering from overweight or anorexia nervosa. Scand J Clin Lab Invest 35:447–454
Lawrence M (1979) Anorexia nervosa: the control paradox. Women's Studies Int Quart 2:91–101
Meddlicott RW (1969) St. Antony Abbot and the hazards of asceticism: an analysis of artists' representations of the temptations. Br J Med Psychol 42:133–140
Palmblad J (1976) Fasting in man. Effects on PMN granulocyte function, plasma iron and serum transferrin. Scand J Haematol 17:217–226
Palmblad J, Fohlin L, Lundstrom M (1977a) Anorexia nervosa and polymorphonuclear granulocyte reactions. Scand J Haematol 19:334–342
Palmblad J, Levi L, Burger A, Melander A, Westgren U, Von Schenk H, Skude G (1977b) Effects of total energy withdrawal (fasting) on the levels of growth hormone, thyrotropin, cortisol, adrenalin, noradrenalin, T4 and T3 in healthy males. Acta Med Scand 201:15–22
Palmblad J, Fohlin L, Norberg R (1979) Plasma levels of complement factors 3 and 4 orosomucoid and opsonic functions in anorexia nervosa. Acta Paediatr Scand 68:617–618
Scrimshaw NS, Taylor CE, Gordon JE (1968) Interactions of nutrition and infection. WHO, Geneva
Smith WR (1969) In: Cox SA (ed) Lectures on the religion of the Semites, 3rd edn. KTAV, New York, pp 443–673 (original 1927)

Stern H (1966) The concept of chastity in biblical society. J Sex Res 2:89–97
Suskind R (1977) Malnutrition and immune response. Raven, New York
Tylor EB (1960) Fasting in the post-biblical period in Sefer Yovel. In: Urbach E (ed) Sefer Yovel for Y. Baer. Erez Israel Society for History and Ethnography, Jerusalem, pp 48–68
Uden AM, Trang L, Venizelos N, Palmblad J (1980) Neutrophil functions and clinical performance after total fasting in patients with rheumatoid arthritis. International Symposia of infections in the immunocompromised Host, Veldhofen, The Netherlands, p 55
Westermerck G (1907) The principles of fasting. Folklore XVIII:403
Westermerck G (1922) The history of human marriage, 5th edn. Allerton, New York

CHAPTER 3

Eating and Eating Behavior

"Leave off first for manner's sake and be not unsatiable, lest thou offend."

Ecclesiastics XXXI 180 B.C.

Since anorexia is a serious aberration of normal eating behavior, it is important to understand the mechanisms of animal and human eating patterns in order to reach a better understanding of the fundamental processes involved in eating. This will be done through an examination of the behavioral and learned eating patterns of animals, as well as the influence of societal, psychological, and cultural factors on both normal and abnormal human eating behavior. Finally the physiological and psychophysiological processes which occur during eating will be examined.

Animal Feeding Behavior

Animal eating behavior is determined by environmental conditions, instinct, and learning. The effect of learned animal eating behavior is especially relevant for a better understanding of human eating patterns. For example, among animals, the mother's behavior will strongly influence the choice of food for the young. When a mother makes a choice of food, even under abnormal conditions, the young will make a similar choice even if the food chosen is bizarre for this species. This is a phenomenon which cannot be easily explained.

In animals *imitative* activity does not seem to be controlled by the same basic laws which govern *instrumental* behavior. Imitative activity occurs in response to a stimulus, normally visual, and the reaction occurs regardless of the reward. If the food consumed brings some desirable sensory input, the reaction may be changed into a typical instrumental response, rewarded by sensory satisfaction. Imitative activity may occur for a long time without such a reward and even when unpleasant feelings develop as a result of the response. Instrumental behavior results from the need to escape from an undesirable sensory state produced by either food deprivation or other factors, to obtain desirable oral satisfaction related to the food consumed, or to obtain other sensory satisfaction not necessarily related to the food eaten.

Animals can respond to artificial sensory input not directly related to food which serves as a reward in feeding. Wyrwicka (1976) showed that rats eat non-nutritional and nonpreferred food after being rewarded by electrical brain stimulation. Cats have been shown to eat bananas for nonoral rewards. It has also been reported that the amount of quinine in food necessary to inhibit eating increased considerably during 54 h of food deprivation in rats. This suggests that food-deprived animals can eat food that is less tasty than that normally accepted.

Eating among animals is also affected by situations of stress and boredom, or it may fill a social function. McGivern and Berntson (1980) showed that in rats stress-induced eating from tail-pinching can be mediated by an increase of endogenous opiates. Since intraventricular administration of beta-endorphin induces eating, and since it was found that naloxone inhibits tail-pinch-induced eating, it appears that stress-induced eating is primarily mediated through an increase in endogenous opiates. Thus in the tail-pinched rat endogenous opiates may be released (due to the discomfort of the pinch) for their analgesic effect, with increased food ingestion being an auxiliary effect. This seems to fit the theory that stress-related hyperphagia is a food-directed manifestation of a more general hyperresponsivity to environmental stimuli (Morley and Levine 1980). Dopamine antagonists like haloperidol may block eating behavior by suppressing growth, which is a prerequisite for ingestive behavior in the rat, whereas naloxone and cholecystokinin (CCK) octapeptide (Muller and Hsiao 1978) appear to produce their effect by inducing satiety without inhibiting growth and licking.

Animals react to psychological stress by exhibiting many behavioral abnormalities, including overeating and fasting. Many stressors may have in common interoceptive stimulus changes, which are sufficiently similar to be indistinguishable from the response selection mechanism, and which therefore elicit responses apparently irrelevant to the particular motivational stage.

Human Eating Behavior

Since humans, in contrast to some animals, cannot store food internally, they have institutionalized and structured their eating patterns so that eating takes place at specific regular intervals (meals). This structuring of eating behavior is determined by social, ethnic, familial, and ecological factors. Also unlike animals, humans have the ability to foresee the future, which has resulted in the development of external storing of food for times of need.

Rozin (1975) analyzed the concept of novelty and familiarity of food, and the conflict between neophobia and neophilia in animals. Food selection, in both animals and humans, seems, among other factors, to be genetically determined. This is shown by the fact that under conditions of stress animals and humans return to familiar food, and Steiner (1973b) found that there seems to be poison avoidance even in the newborn.

As shown in a study by Garb and Stunkard (1974), food aversions among humans most commonly develop in the 6–12 year age range. As with other drive behavior, humans have regulated eating in order to insure that society will have control over this drive. Rituals and rules have been developed so that food cannot be ingested by impulse alone. The time of meals has been set, food is flavored and cooked, and certain food combinations are prohibited. These rituals and taboos have national and religious values and are affected by geographic conditions.

Appetite, in contrast to hunger, is determined by psychologic factors and is less subject to change. The appetite for food is connected with other appetites, such as for sleep and sex. It can be determined by cultural factors, as well as by mood and aesthetics.

Appetite is also a characteristic of certain personality types. Intense people eat intensively. Visceral individuals, who delight in pleasant tastes and smells, eat attentively and with concentration; they take their time to enjoy food through their senses. Individuals who lack development of taste buds eat fiercely, intensively, and with little discrimination. By eating intensively they may desire to either stimulate or fill up the body. The extroverted person, who is easily stimulated by eroticism eats quickly and intensively, coming to speedy climax with both food and sex. There are also individuals whose appetite is insatiable. Immediately after satisfaction they must begin to eat again.

Nevertheless, appetite is a typical human characteristic, one through which needs and drives are expressed, and as such requires a refined sense of discrimination.

Anorectic Eating Behavior

Under normal conditions food has little emotional value, though its social values are manifold. Food plays a large part in family gatherings, festive occasions, and meetings with the opposite sex. In contrast, people with eating disorders invest food with emotional content and associations. In these cases food, essential for life, can be used for motives of rebellion, punishing or killing oneself, withdrawal from others, withholding for purification, and as a means of expressing guilt. Food can also be used as a means of controlling oneself or others.

The female is usually more prone to eating disorders. Obesity seems to be twice as common among women than men, and the rate of anorexia nervosa is at least 12 times as common in the female. Feeding disorders often occur at crucial periods in a woman's life: at puberty, during and after pregnancy, and at menopause. Both a woman's biological/social role and psychological factors may predispose her to eating disorders.

Food and nutrition in general are matters considered to be in the hands of women. The preparation of food is seen as an act of love, of giving, of the gift of life. As mothers, women influence the eating patterns of their children. It is possible that as early as during suckling or bottle-feeding mothers can influence eating behavior.

For women, however, food is also part of the issue of self-control and self-denial. These attributes are seen by society as positive. The search for pleasure is usually seen as a moral weakness. Only in old people, when sexual pleasure is assumed to have decreased, is eating for pleasure commendable and tolerated.

Denial of food has also been seen as a way to deny sexual pleasure and satisfaction in earlier culture patterns. Both sex and the need for food have been considered as sins of the flesh. Asceticism recognizes a duality of body and mind. The corporal part of human nature is considered unclean and connected with inherited sin. It is the unclean body which tries to pull the mind down to the profane. Women's bodies especially are considered unclean and dangerous, as the repository of sexual desires which cause men to sin. Women's bodily functions, especially menstruation, are seen as impure.

As a result, men have tried to control and diminish women's bodies by propagating ideals of feminine beauty which are unrealistic and unhealthy. In the nineteenth century femininity was connected to the ideals of sensitivity, fragility, and physical weakness. In an almost epidemic form, not only fragility but invalidism and chronic illness were the fate of women. A morbid aesthetic existed, in which beauty equaled illness.

These historical views of femininity may be the forerunners of today's epidemic of anorexia nervosa. In both manifestations women are made unrealistic and unable to deal with life. This romantic ideal of a suffering, almost bodiless woman, is certainly the opposite of the type of woman men most feared, the devilish seducer who caused men to sin.

In our own times thinness has replaced the ideal of fragility, though it is a no less unrealistic and destructive ideal. The media portrays successful women as thin. Thin people are considered to be clever and sporty, while fat people are seen as social deviants. All manner of bad qualities are attributed to fat individuals, including stupidity, lack of self-control, impulsiveness, and laziness.

It is through their bodies that women are expected to express themselves and by which their worth is measured, and the bodily ideal which society most values is thinness. This involves the woman in contradictory roles: on the one hand, she is to be the nurturer, giving food to others, while, on the other hand, since the ability to attract men determines a woman's worth, she must deny herself food in order to achieve thinness. It is therefore not surprising that food and body shape is used by women as a means of rebellion. This form of rebellion is also the result of society's expectation of female behavior. The fight for autonomy is unusual in girls. Girls are expected to be quiet and obedient, while boys are permitted to rebel or be aggressive at certain stages. Therefore the process of socialization is different in the sexes, because expectations are different. This in turn means that a girl trying to express her autonomy is already exceptional, and she has to express it in a special way in order to be felt. Society only allows women two forms of expression, either through histrionic dramatic behavior, or through the erotization of the body and behavior.

Regulatory Mechanisms of Food Intake

The onset of depression and anxiety correlates with spasm and the contraction of the muscles of mastication. This is shown by the common practice, before the introduction of anesthesia, of giving the patient something to bite on during surgery. And gum-chewing during examinations seems to have an anxiety-reducing effect.

Mutt (1980) demonstrated that CCK is widely distributed throughout the brain as well as in the gastrointestinal tract. CCK was the first neuropeptide implicated as a putative short-term satiety hormone, which potentially inhibits spontaneous, sham-, and starvation-induced feeding in the rat after peripheral but not central administration (Gibbs et al. 1973). Furthermore, the satiety effect of CCK is abolished by vagotomy, suggesting a peripheral site of action (Louis-Sylvestre and LeMagnen 1980). Bombesin, a tetradecapeptide, is also widely distributed throughout the mammalian brain and gut. Bombesin also suppresses tail-pinch-induced feeding in rats. Corticotropin-releasing factor (CRF) is thought to be the initiator of the general adaptation to stress syndrome as described by H. Selye (1950). CRF suppresses deprivation-induced ingestive behavior. Stress may lead to either under- or overeating. Morley et al. (1983) has pointed out that the anorectic effect of CRF suggests that it is an important candidate peptide for the mediator in stress-induced anorexia.

Straus and Yalow (1979) have suggested that the low levels of CCK reported in the brains of genetically obese mice may be causally related to the hyperphagia present in these animals. Margules et al. (1978) have reported that CCK, TRH and insulin are reported to be satiety factors decreasing food intake, while beta-endorphin has been implicated in states of increased food ingestion. In general, there is controversy as to whether dopamine has a stimulatory or inhibitory role. However, Hemmes et al. (1979) present an intriguing report that the body weight of the genetically obese rats was greatly reduced after long-term ingestion of L-dopa. Grossman (1962) found that intracerebral injection of the adrenergic transmitters norepinephrine (NE) or epinephrine (E) could induce an eating response in fully satiated rats or potentiate the eating response in rats who were already hungry. Slangen and Miller (1969) found that tricyclic antidepressants elicited eating when injected into the medial paraventricular nucleus.

In examining the hyperphagic reaction as a response to stress, experimental findings suggest that this reaction is not primarily a biologically determined phenomenon, but rather a learned response (see for example LeMagnen 1981; LeMagnen et al. 1980). The sensory stimuli to eat, or the palatability of food determines meal size, at least partially through the vagal-mediate cephalic phase of insulin release.

The particular role of the oropharyngeal area, and therefore the sensory activity of food in the overall satiation process has been examined by Rolls et al. (1979). They found that an increase in meal size with successive or simultaneous presentation of various foods (as seen in the currently popular notion of "cafeteria-induced" hyperphagia) results from the fact that both the initial stimulating value and the satiating power of each food item is sensory-stimulus specific rather than nutrient specific. Electrophysiological recordings in the lateral hypothalamic area have demonstrated this sensory specificity of satiation in the monkey.

The role played by gastrointestinal and other factors in satiation, and therefore in determining meal size, is highly controversial (see for example LeMagnen 1981). The action of food on gastric and intestinal mechano- or chemoreceptors and the action of gastrointestinal hormones (for instance CCK) are still obscure (Mutt 1980). Sensory stimuli provided by food passing through the alimentary canal are "conditioned stimuli" for eating and its cessation. Evidence has been presented that from a background of genetically determined preferences and aversions, the overall palatability of each food is conditioned and permanently modulated by the postingestive nutritional effects of the food acting as unconditioned stimuli. Through this conditioning, preferences and aversions are shaped on the basis of sensory qualities, and so the amount eaten of various foods may roughly anticipate their nutritional properties and adjust to current metabolic requirements. The only exception is the hyperphagia induced by high-fat diets (Teixeira et al. 1973). LeMagnen (1981) found that in rats, under ad-lib feeding conditions, the fall of glucose availability and glucose uptake by sensing cells is indeed responsible for the systemic stimulation to eat, or hunger arousal. The exogenous and endogenous supplies of carbohydrates and other metabolites in energy metabolism are the main factors in the maintenance of blood glucose and therefore in the absence of the urge to eat called satiety. No specific satiety-stimulus and no target-site for such a stimulus (claimed for a long time to be in the ventromedial hypothalamus) exist. Unlike the mechanism of active stimuli which abolishes the stimulation to eat at the end of a meal, satiety is a passive state.

As in many other circadian rhythms, darkness and light are only long-term synchronizers of periodic physiological events. Dark and light per se (and hence the suprachiasmatic nuclei) are not the pacemakers. Louis-Silvestre (1976) has shown that rats are hyperinsulinar at night. Both basal and glucose-stimulated insulin release are elevated. Penicaud and LeMagnen (1980) have also shown that tissue sensitivity to insulin (in other words, glucose uptake by tissues under the effect of insulin) is also higher at night than during the day. All the above evidence in favor of the primary role of lipogenesis at night and lipolysis during the day, and of the secondary nature of hyperphagia or hypophagia, give added support to the notion that the pacemaker is associated with mechanisms governing the neuroendocrine metabolic pattern. The onset of successive meals is accelerated at night because the high rate of glucose uptake causes the more frequent occurrence of the slight cytoglucopenia that is the triggering stimulus for eating. During the day, the same stimulation to eat occurs less frequently because the supply of endogenous lipid and carbohydrate metabolites to tissues limits the need and utilization of exogenous carbohydrates for maintaining the blood glucose level.

Evidence has accumulated for a liporegulatory role of the ventromedial hypothalamus (VMH) (see Leibowitz and Rossakis 1979). Obesity after a VHM lesion is primarily due to the disappearance of the neuroendocrine network that directly induces lipolysis and promotes lipogenesis. It has also been seen that the neuroendocrine pattern that brings about lipolysis involves (a) the activation of various descending sympathetic pathways by the VMH direct innervation of the adipose tissues, (b) sympathetic activation of adrenal catecholamine release, (c) splanchnic innervation of the endocrine pancreas (which inhibits insulin and stimulates glucagon release), and finally (d) direct splanchnic innervation of the liver (Frohman and Bernardis 1971).

Thus, there is good support for the view that, in intact rats, the stimulation of the VMH gives rise, via sympathetic activation, to a neuroendocrine state including the inhibition of insulin secretion, which promotes fat mobilization. After a VMH lesion, sympathetic activation is abolished while the parasympathetic innvervation of pancreatic islets is disinhibited and exaggerated, and causes hyperinsulinism. There are also highly glucose-sensitive neurons in the VMH or its vicinity and their glucose sensitivity is insulin dependent (Woods et al. 1979).

Concerning the lateral hypothalamic feeding system, there is support for the notion that the monitoring of feeding is dependent on a neuronal network in which the lateral hypothalamus is a critical site. This site appears to be directly involved in the control of food intake and not in the control of neuroendocrine and metabolic events. Rolls et al. (1976) show that external (olfactory, gustatory, and visual) afferents and presumably visceral afferents project to the lateral hypothalamus and are integrated with blood-borne metabolic signals. There is considerable evidence for the presence of glucose-sensitive and insulin-independent sensors in the lateral hypothalamic area. It is assumed that the glucose-sensitive sites here are stimulated by minimal insulin-independent glucopenia resulting from hypoglycemia, and that this stimulation, associated with the action of sensory afferents, determines feeding patterns. Thus, while the VMH lesion suppresses the nycthemeral periodicity and leaves intact the prandial one, lesion of the lateral hypothalamus retains the former and abolishes the latter. Thus, prandial periodicity is monitored by the lateral hypothalamic system, while its 24 h modulation by the nycthemeral metabolic cycle is controlled by the VMH.

Schlemmer et al. (1979) showed that clonidine, an alpha-noradrenergic agonist, induces profound hyperphagia and subsequent rapid weight gain in macaque monkeys. Clonidine possibly interferes with the central regulation of eating by initially overriding the day-to-day controls detailed by LeMagnen (1981) and then by creating a differently organized feeding pattern.

The question of whether anorectic or bulimic patients are insulin resistant or insulin sensitive is therefore still ambiguous. Before this question can be properly addressed, metabolic, neural, and hormonal signals must be integrated into a logical concept.

Glucostatic Hypothesis

Mayer (1953, 1968) first formulated the glucostatic hypothesis. He postulated that the ventromedial nucleus of the hypothalamus might respond to changes in the rate of glucose utilization and thus regulate food intake. The hypothesis was based on several observations. First, the CNS is known to depend primarily on glucose for its metabolic needs, although it has little capacity to store it and is thus dependent on a continuous supply from the blood. Second, the proportional change in glucose stored as glycogen between meals is much greater than for other substances. Third, the concentration of blood glucose is controlled by several endocrine mechanisms. Fourth, glucose oxidation regulates the oxidation and synthesis of fat.

Many experimental and interpretative lines support this hypothesis (Stunkard and Wolff 1956). Many are indirect indices, but others are direct, for instance, reciprocal electrical activity in the ventromedial and lateral hypothalamus. During periods of hunger and food-seeking, the ventromedial nucleus was electrically inactive, and the lateral area showed increased activity. With satiety, which was associated with high glucose utilization, the VMH was active, and the activity of the lateral hypothalamus was decreased.

Steffens (1969) found that insulin concentrations dropped to low levels just before the onset of a meal. This would be associated with reduced glucose utilization which, according to the glucostatic hypothesis, should initiate eating.

Panksepp (1974) has observed that radioactive glucose is accumulated in greater quantities in the VMH than in the lateral hypothalamus six hours after giving radioactive glucose by stomach tube. The hypothalamus contains cells which accumulate glucose and which may be sensitive to insulin and thus function in the control of stored calories in the body. However, the peripheral glucoreceptors may be just as important as these central mechanisms.

Lipostatic Hypothesis

This lipostatic theory was first proposed by Kennedy (1950, 1953, 1966, 1972) on the basis of studies in rats with injury to the VMH. Initially, free fatty acids were considered to be the metabolic products giving the control signal. Kennedy believes that glycerol is a much better candidate. It is released during the hydrolysis of triglycerides in adipose tissue. This glycerol cannot be reutilized by adipose tissue because a key enzyme, glycerol kinase, is either absent or in very low concentration in this tissue. For this reason, glycerol is released into the circulation in proportion to the rate of hydrolysis of triglycerides. Glycerol in the circulation is transported to the liver, where it can be readily converted into glucose. Such glucose might in turn provide a signal to the hepatic glucoreceptors and hence to the brain. Goodner et al. (1973) found that the hypothalamus metabolizes glycerol more rapidly than does the cortex, but still at a slow rate compared with the liver or kidney. The hypothalamus did not display any special permeability of the blood-brain barrier for glycerol entry. Thus, glycerol remains a possible messenger, either indirectly through glucose formation in the liver or directly through specific glycerol receptors in the hypothalamus (Bray 1976).

Prostaglandins, which are derivatives of arachidic acid are released during lipolysis in adipose tissue. One of them might serve as a messenger, as evidenced by the observations of Martin and Baile (1973), who found that prostaglandin PGE will increase food intake if injected into the hypothalamus of sheep. Had PGE depressed food intake, it would be more consistent with the hypothesis.

Hervey (1969, 1971, 1973) suggested a novel approach to the problem of a signal for the lipostatic mechanism. He proposed a mechanism for sensing the storage of energy, and that totally stored energy is mainly regulated through changes in food intake. The regulatory substance dissolved in the fat must be "sensed" in the CNS. Steroids possibly comprise one such group of regulatory substances. Progesterone is a steroid which will increase body fat.

Thermostatic Hypothesis

Heat production, reflected in changes of body temperature, was proposed by Brobeck (1948, 1960) as a regulator of food intake. This concept is supported by the observation that homoiothermic animals eat more in cold than in hot environments. Several experiments concerning temperature influences on the hypothalamus pointed in the same direction.

Aminostatic Hypothesis

Mellinkoff et al. (1956) observed an inverse relationship between the levels of amino acids and food intake. The receptor system for detecting the deficient amino acid appears to be in the brain. If a small quantity of the deficient amino acid is given into the carotid artery, food intake is not depressed. Experiments have shown that these receptors are most probably not in the VMH.

In order to understand more fully the normal functions which occur during eating we will briefly discuss the organs which are involved in food intake.

Oral Perception: Anatomy, Sensory and Motor Functions, and Their Meanings

The Mouth

The tongue and lips are the only body parts with which humans unknowingly and almost incessantly touch themselves. The tongue in the oral cavity, a closed region, can be said to represent an early model of the world. The human baby, as yet possessing no knowledge of the external world, can nevertheless use its tongue to explore other structures. Spitz (1955) states: "Here probably start all perceptions and the oral cavity therefore has the function of a bridge from the primary reception of stimuli coming from inside the body to external perception." In addition, the contact of the tongue with its oral environment, through the contrast between the mobility of the testing organ and the rigidity of the tested area, seems to make the difference between subject and object conspicuous. The transcendent outer world still remains in limbo. Therefore, the differentiation between tongue and cavity can prepare the infant for the differentiation between subject and object.

The oral cavity is also a microcosmos, symbolizing the body and its basic qualities: wideness, narrowness, direction, tension, swelling, intensity, and rhythm. The closed mouth is a closed cave, while the wide-open mouth is a cave into which streams the cool vastness of the outside world.

In infancy, objects are mouthed and tongued. Spitz (1955) stated that it appears significant that the inside of the mouth, the oral cavity, fulfills the conditions of partaking for perceptive purposes, both on the inside and on the outside. The mouth is simultaneously an interoceptor and an exteroceptor, the oral cavity fulfilling the function of a bridge from internal to external perception. Anorectics can be seen, in some sense, as having regressed to this initial stage of sensory perception by sensing with the mouth only.

The oral cavity, with its equipment of tongue, lips, cheeks, and nasopharynx is the first surface in life to be used for tactile perception and exploration. All perception taking place through the instrumentality of the mouth is still contact perception and thus basically different from distance perception, such as visual and auditory perception. Human communication is built upon both verbal and nonverbal signal systems. The nonverbal system includes mimicking, gestures, and postures. The term verbal communication is used for all signals involving vocalization. All types of human communication are "anthroposemeiotic."

Since the mouth is the primary organ of feeling and satisfaction, it remains an erotogenic zone. Some people, particularly women, smack their lips when experiencing oral or sexual pleasure. Very often the mouth is not only primarily erotogenic, but also closely "imitates" genital play. The mouth is used for sexual acts: kissing, touching other lips as objects, playing with the tongue in another person's mouth, sucking, searching for a way of entering the other's cavity, etc. There is potential swelling of the lips and they get wet, just as the labia of the vagina do. The mouth can therefore be used as a primary pleasure organ for the acting out of sexual feelings. In addition, aggression (both sexual and nonsexual) can be expressed with the mouth by biting, chewing, and grinding of the teeth (bruxism). Yawning, opening the cavity widely towards another person, can also be used as a sign of open aggression, saying, in effect, "you bore me."

There is also complex coordination between the tongue and mandibular muscles in chewing, speaking, swallowing, and other oral actions. The tongue has extrinsic muscles (attached to the skeleton, cranium, and mandible) and intrinsic muscles. These allow the tongue to change shape and form purposefully. The infant uses the tongue in the manipulation of air, and of the nipple and milk. It is also the primary site of empathic linkage between infant and mother. The linkage is implemented at breast-feeding, at nonnutritive suckling, in other interpersonal manipulations of the mouth and head, and when the infant cries or makes other responsive sounds. Variations in infant behavior reflect not only the capacity of the infant to provide cues during feeding, but also the capacity of the nursing mother to respond to cues provided by the infant.

The nonnutritive suckling pattern of human infants is based on rhythmic alternations of bursts and pauses (in contrast to apes). This pattern consists of bursts of 5–20 sucks lasting around 7 s, followed by a nonsucking interval of equal duration.

The development and use of other senses, and their derivative input from the external world, takes place only at a later stage.

Oral Sense

The oral sense was investigated by Ludwig Edinger in 1911. In brain examination he found a very large lobus olfactorius (parolfactorius) in the chameleon and birds. He also noticed that it was the olfactory fibers in the brain which were the first to mature. He then developed a unified concept of smelling, tasting, oral, skin, and mucosa sensorium, which he conceived as a morphologic and functional unit. Furthermore, as von Weizsäcker (1950) proved, sensory functions are always coupled with motor functions. For example, tasting always involves simultaneous chewing, smelling and breathing.

Tellenbach (1968) suggested that during human evolution, with the assumption of an erect posture, vision and hearing became the most important functions, while the oral sense became used for vegetative, digestive, and sexual purposes. A baby, during its first hours of life, reacts to smell and taste stimuli. It is through these senses that it experiences its first contact with the external world.

In contrast to the auditory and visual senses, the sense of smell can only be used for things close by. Smelling can almost be seen as tasting at a distance. However, in order to smell or taste we must first incorporate a substance into our body. The senses of smell and taste are activated when we perform our most basic needs, breathing and eating.

The oral sense also helps to promote a feeling of closeness. From the beginning, the infant uses this sense to differentiate between the known and trustable and the foreign and alien. The breast-feeding mother is a prototype for closeness. This association is later continued through the social use of meals and the sharing of food as a form of becoming intimate with other people.

The oral sensation concerns a substance. In contrast to memories of sensory experiences in the visual or auditory sphere, which are figurative, the memories of smell or taste are limited in time and "evaporate" quickly. Smells or tastes are associated with certain characteristics of objects or parts of objects, but not the whole. We even relate meanings to oral sensations, as can be seen in the expressions "bitter renunciation," "sweet surrender," and "sour effort." As Schippergas (1958) has stated, "Smell creates a milieu for the person, it brings the distance close and brings it to the self. At the same time it keeps distance to the world and relates to the objective. It makes people and things known, brings them close and holds them at a distance."

Concrete sensory experiences can be changed by learning. Tastes can be developed. We can learn to like smells or tastes which might generally be considered as unpleasant. The oral sense can therefore be viewed in part as a learned value, a judgment which can be changed.

Taste Perception

The anatomical basis of taste appears to be, ontogenetically, very old, and taste itself seems to be, phylogenetically, an ancient sense. Taste perception is expressed as a well-differentiated motor reaction of the facial muscles to taste stimuli. It is a rigidly fixed feature of innate character, and is controlled by neural structures of the brainstem. Physical and chemical events originating from either the external or the internal environment of a living organism become sensory stimuli when the organism is equipped with appropriate sensory receptors. These receptors are able to transduce the energetic event and encode it into the language of neural signals. Signals coming from the peripheral receptors become meaningful messages for the organism when the neuronal system is able to decode them and to utilize the sensory input as relevant information. Organisms can respond to a peripheral sensory stimulus by a broad spectrum of reactions. These can involve either the organism as a whole or be related to particular organ systems. Sensory stimuli may be answered by responses which are complex, involving cognitive and psychic processes.

The Implications of These Oral Aspects for Anorexia

In anorectics there is a regression to vegetative control instead of conscious control. This is expressed in the restriction of input by reduced reaction to temperature stimuli to the skin, and reduction of pain sensation. There is also a reduction of metabolic need for calories through reduced peripheral formation of triiodothyronine (T_3) and the attendant mild peripheral hypothyroidism (Vijayan and McCann 1979).

Anorectic individuals report a weaker preference for sweet items, while obese individuals tend to prefer items high in flavor and normal-weight persons like natural-tasting items. Anorectics also seem to exhibit a disturbed awareness of inner processes (Bawkin and Bawkin 1972), which include misperceptions of hunger, satiety, and other bodily sensations such as lack of response to fatigue, cold, pain, and sexual feelings, as well as an interoceptive confusion. One could speculate that there is a regression in the anorectic to sensing by interoception – by tactile sensation in the mouth, which may trigger visual images influenced by tactile elements (body perception).

The anorectic seems to use the body as a substitute for the external environment. Oral perception is increased while proprioception and perception of external stimuli are reduced. This in turn leads to overestimation of object size which can result in a fear of the oversized in general, and therefore the refusal to swallow and incorporate objects that are large. Anorectics also exhibit a fear of changing both size and shape, as well as a fear of loss of control. This fear of loss of control is seen especially in relation to food, which is the stimulus for growth. In the same way, sex is feared on account of pregnancy and its resulting increase in size.

It is interesting to note that many fairy tales center around eating and changes in the body or body parts. These changes usually occur during dreaming or in ecstatic states. Fairy tales express our deepest wishes, fantasies, and fears. The thrill and fascination with growth is universal. All humans experience changes in size, whether through pregnancy, the development of secondary sex characteristics, or pathological growths. These changes are fundamental biological processes and beyond one's power of control. They cannot be stopped and are as irreversible as time itself.

In anorexia, the fear of eating and growing can be a symbolic expression of the fear of biological processes going on without self-control. It is an extreme last effort to fight existence, because existence means growth, separation, and growth once again. These fears may be even more obvious in those individuals where the individuation-separation phase is somewhat arrested. Fear of human contact is such that food, the inanimate, can be turned into the object. For the anorectic, swallowing food may mean not only its incorporation, but also the fusing and resulting internal growth which is so feared. With the object personified in food, the anorectic can, by regulating the amount of food eaten, have complete control over these fears.

To the adolescent, growth, of course, also means differentiation from the neuter, i.e., the differentiation into male or female. While adolescents experience excitement as their bodies change, there is also the fear of the infinite, and of the uncontrollable. This fear can be seen as an expression of the fantasized wish to return to the timelessness of existence and the desire to return to fusion with the mother.

Female anorectics seem to fear the inevitability of change from the undifferentiated child to the individualization of the mature woman. They exhibit a phobia of growing, and therefore avoid eating, consuming only the bare minimum to sustain life. By avoiding the most vital drive, hunger, they are able to convert their helplessness into strength. The sex drive, with its inherent threat of regression and danger of fusion, is also resisted.

Drug Addiction

In common with those suffering from other dyscontrol syndromes, drug addicts exhibit a lack of motivation for treatment and a sense that they cannot be helped. They find relief from unbearable and painful feelings by the incorporation of their objects. There is a reluctance to adopt a sick role. The omnipotence of manipulating bodily feelings belongs to the oral phase of psychosexual development. Drug addicts are brought for treatment by others. They are admitted to the hospital for "withdrawal."

Children play "doctor" out of curiosity and in order to fulfill the need to learn about their differences and identities and to explore erotogenic zones. This is done in secrecy, far from the parental eye. This early sexual play is both a battle for autonomy and an urgent need for satisfaction. It satisfies the need for touch, sight, and adventure. Such infantile hunger and craving remain, never to be wholly satisfied and may be expressed later in life as certain disorders.

The adult addict uses stimuli, manipulating them to delay gratification. We found (Edelstein 1975) that addicts use drugs to satisfy the craving for excitement. Drugs are seen as seductive objects which can either be kept under control or given in to. The thrill of playing with drugs may lead to euphoric or even ecstatic feelings. The omnipotence is shown also in the use of drugs for the opposite effect, namely, for the suppression of feelings, resulting in apathy to oneself and others, as is seen with the use of opioids. It could be a turning of oral tasting pleasure into global somatic pleasure. The addict is able to change internal feelings and perceptions by the use of forces from outside the body.

References

Bawkin H, Bawkin RW (1972) Behavior disorders in children. Saunders, Philadelphia

Bray GA (1976) Peripheral metabolic factors in the regulation of feeding. In: Silverston T (ed) Dahlem workshop on appetite and food intake. Abakon, Berlin, pp 141–176

Brobeck JR (1948) Food intake as a mechanism of temperature regulation. Yale J Biol Med 20:545–552

Brobeck JR (1960) Food and temperature. Recent Prog Horm Res 16:439–459

Dellow PG, Lund JP, Babcock K, Van Rosendall G (1970) The oral assessment of object size. J Speech Hear Res 13(3):526–536

Edelstein EL (1975) Elaborations on the meaning of repetitive behavior in drug-dependent personalities. Br J Addict 70:365–373

Edinger L (1911) Vorlesungen über den Bau der nervösen Zentralorgane des Menschen und der Tiere, 8th edn. Vogel, Leipzig, pp 371–384

Frohman LA, Bernardis LL (1971) Effect of hypothalamus stimulation on plasma glucose, insulin and glucagon levels. Am J Physiol 221:1596–1603

Garb J, Stunkard A (1974) Taste aversions in man. Am J Psychiatry 131:1204–1207

Gibbs J, Young RC, Smith GP (1973) Cholecystokinin elicits satiety in rats with open gastric fistulas. Nature 245:323–325

Goodner CJ, Ogilvie JT, Koerker DT (1973) The metabolism of glycerol by hypothalamic and pituitary tissues in vitro in the rat. Proc Soc Exp Biol Med 143:616–622

Grossman SP (1962) Direct adrenergic and cholinergic stimulation of hypothalamic mechanisms. Am J Physiol 2(2):872–882

Hemmes RB, Pack HM, Hirsch J (1979) Chronic ingestion of L-dopa dramatically reduces body weight of the genetically obese zucker rat. Fed Proc 38:227

Hervey GE (1969) Regulation of energy balance. Nature 22:629–631

Hervey GE (1971) Physiological mechanisms for the regulation of energy balance. Proc Nutr Soc 30:109–116

Hervey GE (1973) Physiological mechanisms in the regulation of energy balance. In: Robertson RF (ed) Anorexia and obesity. Royal College of Physicians, Edinburgh, pp 7–17

Kennedy GC (1950) The hypothalamic control of food intake in rats. Proc R Soc [Biol] 137: 535–549

Kennedy GC (1953) The role of depot fat in the hypothalamic control of food intake in the rat. Proc R Soc [Biol] 140:578–592

Kennedy GC (1966) Food intake, energy balance and growth. Br Med Bull 22:216–220

Kennedy GC (1972) The regulation of food intake. Adv Psychosom Med 7:91–99

Kogure S, Onoda N, Takagi SF (1980) Responses of lateral hypothalamic neurons to odours before and during stomach distension in unanesthetized rabbits. Proceedings of 28th International Congress of Physiological Sciences. International Union of Physiological Sciences

Kram KM, Owen GM (1974) Nutritional studies on US pre-school children: dietary intakes and practices of food procurement, preparation and consumption. In: Fomon SJ (ed) Infant nutrition. Saunders Philadelphia, pp 3–18

LaPointe LL, Williams WN, Hepler EL (1973) Illusion in size perception of intra-orally presented holes. Percept Mot Skills 36:1047–1050
Leibowitz SF, Rossakis C (1979) Mapping studies of brain dopamine-, and epinephrine-sensitive sites, which cause feeding suppression in the rat. Brain Res 172:101–113
LeMagnen J (1981) The metabolic basis of dual periodicity of feeding in rats. Behav Brain Sci 4:561–607
LeMagnen J, Devos M, Larue-Achagiotis C (1980) Food deprivation induced parallel changes in blood glucose, plasma free fatty acids and feeding during the two parts of the diurnal cycle in rats. Neurosci Biobehav Rev 4(1):17–23
Louis-Sylvestre J (1976) Preabsorptive insulin release and hypoglycemia in rats. Am J Physiol 230:56–60
Louis-Sylvestre J, LeMagnen J (1980) Reciprocal interaction between food palatability and vagally mediated preabsorptive insulin release: Suppression of differential food palatability in vagotomized rats. 7th International Conference on the Physiology of Food and Fluid Intake (ICPFFI VII), Warsaw
Margules DL, Moisset B, Lewis MJ, Shibuya H, Pert CB (1978) Beta-endorphin is associated with overeating in genetically obese mice and rats. Science 202:988–991
Martin FH, Baile CA (1973) Feeding elicited in sheep by intrahypothalamic injections of PGE_1. Experientia 29:306–307
Mayer J (1953) Glucostatic mechanism of regulation of food intake. N Engl J Med 249:13–16
Mayer J, Arees EA (1968) Ventromedial glucoreceptor system. Fed Proc 27:1345–1348
McGivern RF, Berntson GG (1980) Mediation of diurnal fluctuations in pain sensitivity in the rat by food intake patterns: reversal by naloxone. Science 210:210–211
Mei N (1978) Vagal glucoreceptors in the small intestine of the cat. J Physiol 282:485–506
Mellinkoff SM, Frankland D, Boyle D, et al (1956) Relationship between serum amino acid concentration and fluctuations in appetite. J Appl Physiol 8:535–538
Morley JE, Levine AS (1980) Stress-induced eating is mediated through endogenous opiates. Science 209:1259–1261
Morley JE, Levine AS, Rowland NE (1983) From minireview: stress-induced eating. Life Sci 32(19):2169–2182
Muller K, Hsiao S (1978) Current status of CCK as a short-term satiety hormone. Neurosci Biobehav Rev 2:79–87
Mutt V (1980) Gastrointestinal hormones. Raven, New York, p 169
Ostreivher HJ, McClure H (1982) A pattern of performance for two age groups of normal adults on a test of oral form discrimination. J Commun Disord 15:329–335
Panksepp J (1974) Hypothalamic regulation of energy balance and feeding behavior. Fed Proc 33:1150–1165
Penicaud L, LeMagnen J (1980) Aspects of the neuroendocrine bases of the diurnal metabolic cycle in rats. Neurosci Biobehav Rev 4(1):39–42
Rolls ET, Burton MJ, Mora F (1976) Hypothalamic neuronal responses associated with the sight of food. Brain Res 111:53–66
Rolls ET, Roper-Hall A, Sanghera MK (1979) The latency of activation of neurons in the lateral hypothalamus and substantia innominata during feeding in the monkey. Brain Res 164:121–135
Rossell HR (1960) The encyclopedia of witchcraft and demonology. Crown, New York
Rozin P (1975) Psychobiological and cultural determinants of food choice. In: Silverstone T (ed) Dahlem workshop on appetite and food intake. Abakon, Berlin, pp 285–312
Schippergas H (1957) Übersetzungen und Erläuterungen zu Texten aus Hildegard von Bingen: Das Buch vom Grund und Wesen und der Heilung der Krankheiten (causae et curae). Müller, Salzburg
Schlemmer RF Jr, Casper RC, Narasimhachari N, Davis JM (1979) Clonidine-induced hyperphagia and weight gain in monkeys. Psychopharmacology (Berlin) 61:233–234

Seyle H (1950) The physiology and pathology of exposure to stress. Actlin, Montreal
Slangen JL, Miller NE (1969) Pharmacological tests for the function of hypothalamic NE in eating behavior. Physiol Behav 4:543–552
Spitz RA (1955) The primal cavity: a contribution to the genesis of perception and its role for psychoanalytic theory. Psychoanal Study Child 10:215–240
Spitz RA (1955–56) Die Urhöhle. Psyche (Stuttg) 9:641–667
Steffens AB (1969) Blood glucose and FFA levels in relation to the meal pattern in the normal rat and the VMH hypothalamic lesion rat. Physiol Behav 4:212–225
Steiner JE (1973a) The human gustofacial response. In: Bosma JF (ed) Fourth symposium on oral sensation and perception: development in the fetus and infant. DHEW publication no (NIH) 73–546
Steiner JE (1973b) The gustofacial response: observations on normal and anencephalic newborn infants – fourth symposium on oral sensation and perception (development in the fetus and infant). In: Bosman JF (ed) DHEW publication no (NIH) 73–546. Fogarty Internat Center Proc 21:254–278
Steiner JE, Rosenthal-Zifrone E, Edelstein EL (1969) Taste perception in depressive illness. Isr Ann Psychiatry 7(2):223–232
Straus E, Yalow RS (1979) Cholecystokinin in the brains of obese and non-obese mice. Science 203:68–69
Stunkard AJ, Wolff HC (1956) Studies on the physiology of hunger: the effect of intravenous administration of glucose on gastric hunger contractions in man. J Clin Invest 35:954–963
Teixeira VL, Antunes-Rodrigues J, Migliorini RH (1973) Evidence for centers in the central nervous system that selectively regulate fat mobilization in the rat. J Lipid Res 14:672–677
Tellenbach H (1968) Geschmack und Atmosphäre (neues Forum). In: Revers WJ (ed) Das Bild des Menschen in der Wissenschaft, vol 8. Müller, Salzburg
Thoman EB, Barnett CR, Leiderman PH (1971) Feeding behavior of newborn infants as a function of parity of the mother. Child Dev 42:1471–1483
Vijayan E, McCann SM (1979) Suppression of feeding and drinking activity in rats following intraventricular injection of thyrotropin-releasing hormone (TRH). Endocrinology 100: 1727–1730
Weizsäcker V von (1950) Der Gestaltkreis. Thieme, Stuttgart
Williams WN, La Pointe LL (1971) Intra-oral recognition of geometric forms by normal subjects. Percept Motor Skills 32:419–426
Woods SC, Lotter EC, McKay LD, Porte D Jr (1979) Chronic intracerebroventricular infusion of insulin reduces food intake and body weight of baboons. Nature 282:503–505
Wyrwicka W (1976) Problem of motivation in feeding behavior. In: Novin D, Wyrwicka W, Bray G (ed) Hunger: basic mechanisms and clinical implications. Raven, New York

CHAPTER 4

The Concept of Body Image and Its Changes

"What is meant by ascetic ideals? ... In women at best, an additional implement of seduction, a little morbidezza on a fine piece of flesh, the anglehood of a plump, pretty animal."

F. W. Nietzsche: The Genealogy of Morals III, 1887

Observations and Examinations

One of the most characteristic features of anorectics is their distorted body image. This feature was noticed as early as over a century ago by Lasegue (1873) who stated: "Patient said she was neither changed nor is she thinner." In more recent times Bruch (1962) talked about distorted inner image as pathognomonic. In 1973 she elaborated on three key symptoms: "A disturbance of delusional proportions in the body image and body concept, a disturbance in the accuracy of perception (or cognitive interpretation) of stimuli arising in the body, and finally, a paralyzing sense of ineffectiveness." How is body image and the anorectic's denial or perceptual distortion to be understood?

Infants are born naked. Slowly the body is explored by touching and later by looking and playing with body parts. The body is simultaneously first object and subject. As the first object it is under constant observation. Later, when clothing is provided, infants include the clothing as belonging to their bodies.

The separation between self and others, between subject and external object after separation from the symbiotic mother relationship, occurs as a natural developmental phenomenon and has been duly described. However, the inclusion of, or separation from clothing has very rarely been mentioned. As subject and object are often not completely separated, the limits of body and nonbody are not always clear. Most of the time our bodies are covered by materials which may be somehow animated. People in general, young or adult, do spend much time, thought, and energy on their bodily appearance. This may be manifested in the striving to develop a certain bodily form as well as being expressed through clothing and hairstyles.

Whatever comes into contact and is an extension of our skin can be included and incorporated into our body scheme. Body image is an abstraction that is difficult to define, but in general terms it may be described as a mental image of the body, a neural representation of it, or the individual's pictorial representation of appearance. In any case, it is basically the idea we have of how our body appears to others. There are, of course, many differences between the ideal we have in our minds of how we would like to look and our actual appearance as we appear to others, and as we think others see us. There is also a difference between our own ideal of how we would like to look and how we feel we look at certain times or moments, especially during some crisis.

"Body awareness" and "body identity" are not limited to "body image," but extend to perception and interpretation of interoceptive stimuli. These may belong to misinterpretation of awareness of inner functions and processes. "Self-image" is the view that the individual has of himself at a particular time in a specific situation. It consists of body image and the representation of the inner state at that time.

At various times in human individual evolution the image of the body, both as a whole or in part, takes on special symbolic importance. This shows us that the concept of body image is not always fixed but may change due to developmental phases or individual crises, for instance due to real, induced, or phantasized changes in body parts. This may also be induced by wishful or magical thinking, as may be the case in anorexia. These ectodermal functions can be seen in the fact that both women and men in certain life phases, and to certain degrees, owe much of their self-image to what they may add or subtract in order to keep to their idealized body image in their daily life. For instance, skin, the outer-most layer of our appearance, is treated with soap, cosmetics, perfumes, and other items which may contribute both to the image as well as to other bodily functions, such as erotic stimulation of the self or others. Sport may be used as a means of developing a certain bodily look. These actions are carried out to promote an image of how we would like to look in order to be more loved. Acceptability to ourselves can also be affected by changes in other aspects of the body appearance such as facial and head hair. In times of crises of psychosocial significance, certain organs of the body may be invested with more cathexis, overvalued, and therefore much scrutinized. This can be seen especially in adolescents' crises, in which one finds special attention being paid to organs symbolizing growth or possible retardation of growth. For example, the nose is considered a symbolic expression of manhood, of symmetry and prowess. The size of the penis is often minimized in adolescents because of internal conflicts and feelings of rejection. The development of breasts and hips in girls can equally disturb hitherto stable development. These conflictual attitudes and disturbances of body image can even be carried over into adulthood, as can be seen from the great numbers of women who have their bust size or shape altered by plastic surgery.

The appearance of certain parts of the body can also arouse feelings of inhibition, ambivalence, and expressions of shame. These feelings are expressions of the transition between the ideal and the real, as, for example, when the adolescent undresses and stands naked in front of a mirror in order to compare the real body to the fantasized body self.

Our observation is that the more disturbed a person is by the size or asymmetry in the overvalued body part the more intervention is used. This particular body part is sensed as deviant, as being disparate from the ideal (whose form depends on the severity of the individual's disturbance). Intervention can mean anything from discussing the problem with others, requesting medical advice and changes, to the psychotic act of interfering with one's body integrity, such as in self-mutilation.

It is by looking and being looked at, the escape into darkness when the body can be hidden or the freedom of light and exposure, that determines much of the body image and how that image connects with self-acceptance and the ability to be close to another human being. Therefore, the possibility of the actualization of a relationship with another person is dependent on a stable body image. One is more able to be intimate both with one's own body and the body of another person the more agreement or closeness there is with one's stable body image. By exposing oneself to intimacy one faces the gap between idealized and real body image, which demands the security or ego-strength to deal with this dichotomy.

There are distortions of certain body areas which we are not able to control, such as oral perception, which usually exaggerates the size of the items in our oral cavity (probably because of ontogenetic historical reasons). Interesting changes in body feeling and body image also occur when using drugs. These include feelings of depersonalization and derealization and a blurring of the distinct boundaries between the body and the outer world. This in turn can produce a change in perceived body image.

It can be assumed that the extension of other sense modalities may also have a determining influence on one's body image, like the extension of clothing. The senses can be used to integrate an attitude of one's whole body, somewhat like a blind person trying to compose an inner image of how an object looks by feeling certain parts. Smell might have something to do with this extension of kinesthetic, tactile stimuli.

Instability in body image, naturally induced changes, or a wide gap between the ideal and the actual can induce severe difficulties in relating both to oneself and others. Anorectics specifically seem to have difficulty with their identity formation and dynamic development. It is for this reason that anorectics express a deviant attitude toward their bodies, especially those parts which are inherently female. Psychologic growth in adolescence is effected by the growth of the secondary sexual characteristics. Breasts, hips, hair, menstruation, belly, etc. all have specific significance. These young women are frequently heard making comments such as: "the belly should be completely flat, or even concave; hips should be more narrow, they are too wide (feminine); my thighs should not touch each other, there should be a distance between them; legs should be really thin."

Anorectics seem to have distortions of perception, or of perceptual awareness, mainly in the perception of their body or body parts (Crisp and Kalucy 1974). They usually complain that they are either too obese or that they look quite normal even when very emaciated. This type of disturbance also includes a conceptual disturbance, which has its base in cognitive and affectual components. There is at some level an awareness that their real size is being wrongly interpreted. Formally this could be related to denial, negative hallucinations, and delusional thinking. Magical thinking, primary process thinking, and other regressive phenomena also effect human cognition, and in turn hamper development. Magical thinking about changes and the growth of certain organs are often mentioned in fairy tales. The infantile mind is busy with fantasies about its own oscillations, with wishes, threats, and anxieties about body changes. In fairy tales, animals are changed into human beings (the frog actually being the prince, who regains his original form after sleeping with the princess), people are changed into beasts, or swallowed by them.

Various changes in body image and body feelings can also be caused by two other syndromes which we have described as dyscontrol syndromes: obesity and drug abuse. Obesity is the expression of an ambivalence towards one's own body, the wide gap between the ideal and the actual, and the anxiety that results from this gap. On the other hand, obesity is also an indication of self-induced shame, and thereby the achievement of another not always obvious aim, namely, the distancing from or avoidance of human contact. The use of drugs and hallucinogens definitely causes disturbed body image perceptions and actual distortions, which become more conscious than with anorexia or obesity. With drug use body boundaries may vary considerably and sometimes, as with functional psychoses, the boundaries between the inner and outer world and the body and other objects become completely confused. It is interesting to note that the schizophrenic person may severely distort his or her body awareness and image. As is done with the surrounding world, primary thinking and other deviations can cause the subjective feeling to be falsified, and body parts, used as symbols, may be misused, split off, and bizarrely distorted. Often their distortion is in *pars pro toto* logic.

The reasons for the distorted body image of the adolescent anorectic are varied (Casper 1981). Do they distort their body image because adolescence is such a critical ambiguous period of life? In addition, do they distort consciously or is anorexia an encapsulated psychotic trait? Bruch (1973) theorizes that the anorectic's characteristic features of weight phobia, self-imposed starvation, and denial of thinness reflect defects in ego-structure that underpin body image, cognitive representation of interoceptive processes, and self-directed autonomy. Goodsitt (1977) claims a faulty development of intrapsychic structures that regulate bodily and self-perceptions. Palazzoli (1978) believes it is symbiotic merging that predisposes the body to self-identity distortions. Thinness may have some symbolic-pictorial meaning, since by occupying such little space one runs no risk of colliding, or fusing with others. And finally, Blatt and Wild (1976) state that "The ontogeny of boundary development involves increasing differentiation between self and non-self, between inner experience and external perceptions, and between independent objects." From these studies it seems conclusive that a marked component of the behavior of anorectics is a disturbed body image.

Some authors have related specifically to the problem of the development of the body image and body size perception. Daurat-Hmjelak et al. (1966) examined the problem of the development of the body ego in children, and found that this development, in the sense of Piaget, reflects the evolution of intellectual abilities. Faterson and Witkin (1970) developed a longitudinal study focusing on the development of the body concept from childhood to adulthood as measured through the technique of human figure drawing. They found that the articulation of the body concept rises sharply from the 8th year to the age of 14, and after that changes only slightly. So that by early adolescence a relative stability of differentiation of the body concept is reached. Gellert (1962) widened this direction of research, trying to understand how (and if) the development of the aspect of the *inner* body is conceptualized. He demonstrated that it was intellectual development which quantitatively and qualitatively decided the picture of the inner parts of the body.

Another interesting aspect of body image can be explored by using cathexis, as used in psychoanalysis, and introducing body cathexis. This measures the gratification which individuals feel for their body parts or their whole body. This instrument developed by Witkin et al. (1962) is called the "Sophistication of Body Concept Scale." This test includes the drawing of a female person and is scored for degree of differentiation. In the work of Strober et al. (1979), this test, together with others, was used. His study showed that anorectics demonstrated less differentiation in their human figure drawings. In our own studies, we asked patients to draw themselves and their mother. From these pictures it was possible to differentiate between two mother-type figures: one a very giving, very feminine mother with large breasts, and the other, usually in the more severe cases, a mother figure which looked completely undifferentiated, neither man nor woman, like a very little boy or girl.

Darby (1970) had the interesting idea, which is important to mention in this context, of letting schizophrenics attend to their own bodies to try to improve their body/outer world boundaries. One group did physical exercises, while the other group only imagined doing so. The result was examined in the Rorschach responses. There were very significant rises in B-responses (barrier) in those who participated in exercises in contrast to preexercise levels. This seemed to suggest that body boundaries can be better developed when attention is given to the body by planned movement and training. Other authors, such as Fisher and Cleveland (1958) found that adaptability to stress caused by severe illness is better in persons with fixed body image boundaries (high B-responses) than those with unstable boundaries. The B-response seemed a particularly good instrument for predicting how adaptability to invalidity will be formed.

White and Wash (1965) measured body cathexis in male and female adolescent students and found that body cathexis and interest show a high correlation with the grade of self-content, with self-assurance, and with anxiety about the body, as well as being learned attitudes from the parents concerning body and self. Kurtz (1969), who also examined students, found the following male-female differences: Women like their own bodies more than men like theirs, are more interested and more observant of their bodies and also have a more differentiated notion of them. Jourard and Secord (1955) measured preestimated ideas of women concerning their body parts. He found that self-estimates of weight and hip-size were significantly smaller than actual measurements, while the estimate of ideal breasts was larger than the actual measurements. Nevertheless, while draw-a-person tests certainly have a fascinating aspect in their various forms of projective ability and are of clinical value, they are not easy to evaluate and do not easily lend themselves to comparative statistical analyses.

Perceived body image may lie close to, or be quite distant from, subjective or objective reality. Interdependent of body image is the problem of ego boundaries, their rigidity, flexibility, uncertainty, instability, fragility, and how penetrable they may be. Rorschach and Holtzmann responses were used in the past to understand the projection of boundary strengths or weaknesses. Much experience in interpreting Rorschach responses has been gathered during the many years of using these highly valued tests. Strober and Goldenberg (1981), using this technique, succeeded in showing more intrusion of both affective and descriptive content in anorectic Rorschach perceptions, a loss of internal/external boundaries, and also a trend toward more deviant conceptual boundary organization, even when compared to depressed controls. Kiener (1974) introduced the idea of using and categorizing germane Rorschach responses, which has since been taken over by other research groups. Well-defined and stable body boundaries were designated as B-responses (barrier). Weakness, lack of substance and of penetrability were designated as P-responses (penetration).

A variety of techniques have been developed to assess body image more scientifically. In the beginning a distorting mirror or a distorting photographic technique was used, such as a projected photograph which could be distorted along the horizontal axis. This procedure involves using an anamorphic lens to distort a slide-photograph of the subject by up to 20% in both directions (under- and overestimation). The patient must then select the image which corresponds best with his current view of his body (on the horizontal axis). This technique was first used by Glucksman and Hirsch (1969), and subsequently, by Garner, Garfinkel and colleagues (Garner et al. 1976; Garfinkel et al. 1977, 1978, 1979) in studies with anorectic patients.

Similar to these techniques and in accordance with recent developments, the distorting television image was developed (Allebeck et al. 1974). It involves using an on-line TV image-distortion procedure, the task of the subjects being to alter the image to correspond with their current view of themselves.

In all these tests, there was overestimation by many of the anorectic patients, but not by the mothers when estimating their daughters. General findings have shown that anorectics markedly overestimate the size of their body parts compared with controls (Pierloot and Hauben 1978). As was found in some of our yet unpublished experiments, anorectics of longer duration will overestimate tactile oral perception of food particles when compared with visual size estimates and with controls. Studies using the above-mentioned techniques and estimates of body parts have found overestimation to be a strong predictor of poor prognosis (Garfinkel et al. 1977).

In the distorting photograph technique (DPT) mentioned above, no clear-cut results could be obtained, although certain studies found that about half of all anorectics showed a marked tendency to overestimate and this was positively related to measures of introversion and lack of self-control. Meerman (1983) found in the television distorting image technique that both anorectic and normal control underestimated their frontal and profile images, with controls underestimating significantly more than anorectics. Studies with the same technique by Freeman et al. (1984) found that anorectics and bulimics overestimated their frontal body size more than controls, while bulimics alone overestimated their profile shape more than all other groups.

Other measurements of body image include:

1. *Visual Size Estimation* (VSE). VSE was originally designed by Slade and Russel (1973). Casper et al. (1979) used it in a modified form.
2. *Size Estimation Technique.* The "prototype size estimation" procedure was developed by Reitman and Cleveland (1984) (the moving caliper technique).
3. *Image-Marking Procedure (IMP) Studies.* A simpler method, called the "image-marking procedure" (IMP), has been described by Askevold (1975) and used in subsequent studies. It involves the patients facing a wall and marking their perceived body width on a sheet of white paper attached to the wall.

It was found that although both anorectic and neurotic controls overestimated their body width, the anorectic on average did so to a significantly greater degree than controls ($T=2, 60$, $P>0.05$). Casper et al. (1979) stated that "although overestimation of body width and depth is a common phenomenon in the young female population, and not limited to anorexia nervosa, the degree of the body image distortion in the individual anorectic patient is related to the severity of the illness and has value as a predictor of weight gain. It also suggested that a psychologic defense mechanism such as denial plays a role in the conceptual integration of body image in anorexia nervosa."

An interesting experiment was made concerning "demand characteristics." It explored how the subjects related to and interpreted instructions, and especially the way they attempted to guess the experimenter's hypothesis. This was shown by Orne, as early as 1969, to be an important factor in experiments of this sort (Orne 1969).

Norris (1984) requested subjects to reestimate their body size after looking in a mirror. It was found that they clearly reduced their overestimation following the initial estimation. The latest experiment in this direction was that of Proctor and Morley (1986) in which 24 patients with anorexia nervosa and 30 normal controls were asked to estimate their body size several times, each time using different instructions. The degree of overestimation was found to vary predictably with the wording of the instructions. Informing the subject that she had made an error, without specifying the direction of the error, resulted in reduced overestimation on a subsequent trial, both for anorectics and controls. "Internally directed" instructions were associated with a greater degree of overestimation than "external" instructions in both groups, but particularly in anorectic subjects. (Internal instructions meant that the subject should estimate her body relying on how she felt her body to be, while the so-called external instructions required the subject to estimate her body size as if she were another person looking at her.)

Other methods make use of a more combined approach and explore wider areas of self-concept, in order to find specificity in the anorectic group. For instance, using the "Ofer Self Image Questionnaire" (Casper et al. 1981) measures the wide area of self-concept of adolescents and found among anorectic girls a predominance of distressing affect, a poor self concept, insecurity in social relationships, and a sense of inadequacy in approaching sexual issues. A wider application of the Casper and Ofer tests is seen in the work of Swift et al. (1986), in which they used two measurements of self concept, the "Ofer Self Image Questionnaire" and the "Structural Analysis of Social Behavior-Introject." The results of these researchers were as follows: Anorectics displayed more psychologic distress than normal controls, the older age group (with a longer duration of illness) demonstrated poorer adjustment, and probably the most significant and interesting finding was that the anorectics had a very high level of self-attack, or, as they called it, a very high level of hostility turned upon the psychological self. These findings fit in well with our own clinical impression of what we call moral masochism and tendency to asceticism. Leon et al. (1985) checked on sexual, body image, and personal attitudes and found significant problem areas in the anorectic group centering on negative feelings about sexuality and body state, a poor self-image, unfavorable evaluation of personality and social-skill abilities, and a lack of confidence and comfort in social situations.

All these various conflicting hypotheses by researchers on the possible psychologic causes of anorexia are the result of using different procedures based on different assumptions, and of using various techniques. The best evaluations seem to be obtained from those procedures which use various techniques of whole body size and body parts' estimates, together with questionnaires. After years of testing, it is possible to produce comparative studies. Fichter et al. (1986) recently compared three different procedures in a discriminant function analysis: a video-monitor procedure, the movable caliper procedure, and the image-marking procedure. The image-marking procedure showed the best discrimination between groups. Anorectic patients showed a statistically significant overestimation as compared with the control group in the variables "waist," "upper thigh," and the compound measure "soft body parts." A standard liquid meal of 240 calories had no statistically significant influence on the estimation of body width.

One of the more recent, interesting, and widely based tests using identity structure analysis (ISA) was conducted by Weinreich et al. (1985). The study was based on three major theoretical orientations (psychodynamic theory, symbolic interactionist perspective of the situated self, and personal construct psychology). The first experimental findings were in agreement with the notion of a common constellation of identity characteristics in anorexia and bulimia, the most salient of these being devalued self-images and conflicts in identification with maternal metaperspectives.

Wingate and Christie (1978), using the Minnesota Multiphasic Personality Inventory (MMPI), have reported that overestimation in anorectics is negatively correlated with ego strength as measured by the E-scale of the MMPI. And finally, reliability studies have been conducted by Gardner and Garfinkel (1981, 1982), by Freeman et al. (1984), and Slade (1985). Slade suggests that the differences in findings between size estimation and image-distorting procedures are qualitative in nature. Image-distorting procedures, he claims, reflect a relatively fixed, cognitive attitude to body size, in other words, a delusional belief. However, size estimation error is thought to be a reflection of a fluid state of body size sensitivity, which is influenced by affective factors. Anorectic subjects, in contrast to controls, displayed a significant correlation in body size estimates from one year to the next. The lack of correlation in body size estimates in normal women is a curious finding and may suggest that normally one's perception of one's size may be quite fluid and complexly determined. The interoceptive disturbance is shown by the "aversion to sucrose test" procedure. This disturbance is also stable from year to year. (Normal subjects rated the taste of sucrose solution as aversive or unpleasant after ingesting a glucose load. Anorectic subjects, in contrast, do not experience any difference in the rated pleasantness of sucrose tastes before as compared with after glucose ingestion). It is interesting to note that significant weight gain did not alter the aversion test of anorectics.

Anorectics are less responsive than normal subjects to internal cues related to nutritional requirements and they may be unable to habituate to repeated exposure to carbohydrate-containing food (Garfinkel et al. 1979). Body image distortions seem related to a lower threshold of sensitivity to undesired body changes.

Summary

In this chapter we have tried to show developmental aspects of the formation of body image. It was shown that body image distortions do in fact exist in the anorectic syndrome and make up a major part of its behavioral aspect. The development of body image has aroused a great deal of interest in the scientific community. Behavioral scientists find it fascinating to build hypotheses and develop sets of measurement, in particular for such forms of deviant appearance as those found in anorectic girls. We shall return to further clarification of this topic when we explore psychodynamic aspects.

References

Allebeck P, Hallberg D, Espmark S (1976) Body image – an apparatus for measuring disturbances in estimation of size and shape. J Psychosom Res 20:583–589

Askerold F (1975) Measuring body image. Psychother Psychosom 26:71–80

Blatt SJ, Wild CM (1976) Schizophrenia: a developmental analysis. Academic, New York

Bruch H (1962) Perceptual and conceptual disturbances in anorexia nervosa. Psychosom Med 24:187–199

Bruch H (1973) Eating disorders: obesity, anorexia nervosa, and the person within. Basic Books, New York

Casper R, Casper C, Halmi KA, Goldberg SC, Eckert ED, Davies JM (1979) Disturbances in body image estimation as related to other characteristics and outcome in anorexia nervosa. Br J Psychiatry 134:60–66

Casper RC, Ofer D, Ostrov E (1981) The self-image of adolescents with acute anorexia nervosa. J Pediatr 98 (4):656–661

Crisp AH, Kalucy RS (1974) Aspects of the perceptual disorder in anorexia nervosa. Br J Med Psychol 47:349–361

Darby JA (1970) Alteration of some body image indexes in schizophrenics. J Consult Clin Psychol 35:116–121

Daurat-Hmeljak C, Stambak M, Berges J (1966) Une epreuve de schema corporel. Rev Psychol Appl 16:141–185

Faterson HF, Witkin HA (1970) Longitudinal study of development of the body concept. Dev Psychol 2:429–438

Fichter MM, Meister I, Koch HJ (1986) The measurement of body image disturbances in anorexia nervosa: experimental comparison of different methods. Br J Psychiatry 148 (4):453–461

Fisher S, Cleveland SE (1958) Body image and personality. Dover, New York

Freeman RJ, Thomas CD, Solyom L, Hunter MA (1984) A modified video-camera for measuring body image distortions: technical description and reliability. Psychol Med 14: 411–416

Garfinkel PE, Moldofsky H, Garner DM, Stancer HC, Coscina DV (1977) Prognosis in anorexia nervosa as influenced by clinical features: treatment and self-perception. Can Med Assoc J 117:1041–1045

Garfinkel PE, Moldofsky H, Garner DM, Stancer HC, Coscina DV (1978) Body awareness in body image and satiety. Psychosom Med 40:487–497

Garfinkel PE, Moldofsky H, Garner DM (1979) The stability of perceptual disturbances in anorexia nervosa. Psychol Med 9:703–708

Garner DM, Garfinkel PE (1981–82) Body image in anorexia nervosa measurement, theory and clinical implications. Int J Psychiatry Med 11(3):263–283

Garner DM, Garfinkel PE, Stancer HC, Moldofsky MD (1976) Body image disturbance in anorexia nervosa and obesity. Psychosom Med 28:327–337

Gellert E (1962) Children's conceptions of the content and functions of the human body. Genet Psychol Monogr 65:293–405

Glucksman ML, Hirsch J (1969) The response of obese patients to weight reduction: the perception of body size. Psychosom Med 31:1–7

Goodsitt A (1977) Narcissistic disturbances in anorexia nervosa. In: Feinstein SC, Giovachini P (eds) Adolescent psychiatry, vol 5. Aronson, New York

Jourard SM, Secord PF (1955) Body cathexis and personality. Br J Psychol 46:130–138

Kiener F (1974) Untersuchungen zum Körperbild (body image). 2. Teil. Z Klin Psychol Psychother 22(1):45–66

Kurtz RM (1969) Sex differences and variations on body attitudes. J Consult Clin Psychol 33:625–629

Lasègue C (1873) De Daurore hystérique. Archives genérales de médicine 21:385–403

Leon GR, Lucas AR, Colligan RC, Ferdinande RJ, Kamp J (1985) Sexual body image and personality attitudes in anorexia nervosa. J Abnorm Child Psychol 13(2):245–258

Meerman R (1983) Experimental investigation of disturbances in body image estimation in anorexia nervosa patients and ballet and gymnastics pupils. Int J Eating Dis 2:91–100

Norris DL (1984) The effects of mirror confrontation on self-estimation of body dimensions in anorexia nervosa, bulimia and two control groups. Psychol Med 14:835–842

Orne MT (1969) Demand characteristics and the concept of quasi-controls. In: Rosenthal R, Rosnow RL (eds) Artifacts in behavioral research. Academic, New York

Palazzoli MS (1978) Self starvation. Jason Aronson, New York

Pierloot RA, Houben ME (1978) Estimation of body dimensions in anorexia nervosa. Psychol Med 8:317–324

Proctor L, Morley S (1986) Demand characteristics in body size estimation in anorexia nervosa. Br J Psychiatry 149:113–118

Reitman EE, Cleveland SE (1964) Changes in body image following sensory deprivation in schizophrenic and control groups. J Abnorm Soc Psychol 68:168–176

Slade PD (1985) A review of body image studies in anorexia nervosa and bulimia nervosa. J Psychiatr Res 19(2/3):255–265

Slade PD, Russell GFM (1973) Awareness of body dimensions in anorexia nervosa: cross-sectional and longitudinal studies. Psychol Med 3:188–199

Strober M, Goldenberg I (1981) Ego boundary disturbance in juvenile anorexia nervosa. J Clin Psychol 37:433–438

Strober M, Goldenberg I, Green J, Saxon J (1979) Body image disturbance in anorexia nervosa during the acute and recuperative phase. Psychol Med 9:695–701

Swift WJ, Bushnell NJ, Hanson P, Logemann T (1986) Self-concept in adolescent anorectics. J Am Acad Child Psychiatry 25(6):826–835

Weinreich P, Doherty J, Harris P (1985) Empirical assessment of identity in anorexia and bulimia nervosa. J Psychiatr Res 19:297–302

White WF, Wash JA (1965) Prediction of successful college academic performance, from measures of body cathexis, self-cathexis and anxiety. Percept Mot Skills 20:431–432

Wingate BA, Christie MJ (1978) Ego strength and body image in anorexia nervosa. J Psychosom Res 22:201–204

Witkin HA, Dyk RB, Faterson HF, Goodenough DR, Karp SA (1962) Psychological differentiation. Wiley, New York

CHAPTER 5

Biological Aspects

Brain Monoamines and Neuropeptides in Relation to Nutrition

After having discussed local mechanisms of food intake and the central mechanisms in charge of hunger and appetite, we will now discuss organic brain aspects.

Anorexia, as well as a whole spectrum of other disorders, involves excessive drive behavior and the compulsive control of it at various levels. Similar "on and off" mechanisms seem to take place in the biological sphere, as correlates of the behavioral aspects. Some biochemical findings in various brain areas hint at inhibitory mechanisms, while others disinhibit even at various circadian rhythms.

It can be shown that a large number of the biological symptoms of anorectics result entirely from minimal food intake and the starvation syndrome. Other symptoms, however, seem to be primary and quite independent of the state of malnutrition, and relate to: increased cortisol production rate, decreased norepinephrine (NE) concentration in the cerebrospinal fluid (CSF), insulin resistance, decreased growth hormone release response to L-dopa, and, finally, an immature circadian pattern for luteinizing hormone secretion (Katz et al. 1978; Kaye et al. 1980; Crisp et al. 1967; Halmi 1978; Katz et al. 1976; Garfinkel 1984).

All the above-mentioned symptoms are at least partially independent of the malnutritive state. For this reason it is believed that a primary hypothalamic functional disorder may be the result or the correlate of a primary psychiatric disorder. It is accepted that stress can alter hypothalamic function together with a whole network of other diencephalic structures, such as the amygdala.

When dealing with the hypothalamus we should be aware that the same and adjacent areas of the hypothalamus regulate feeding, menstrual activity, sexual behavior, temperature and pain sensation. Since all these functions are disturbed in anorectics, many researchers are prone to see anorexia nervosa as the expression of hypothalamic disease (Bray and York 1979; Ban 1966). The hypothalamus also has a primary influence over the autonomic nervous system. However, the hypothalamus is also believed to be the regulator of many afferent impulses, emotional stimuli, and motivated behavior, and may therefore act as one of several integrating factors.

There is some evidence that, in general, the medial hypothalamus exerts a tonic sympathetic control over visceral functions whereas the lateral hypothalamus exerts a parasympathetic effect. Teitelbaum and Epstein (1962) and Grossman (1975) showed that, when looking for a model of anorexia, starvation syndrome in animals could be produced by lateral hypothalamus lesions. Animals with such inflicted lesions neither eat nor react to stimuli and may starve to death. If there is only slight neural damage, or if there has been time for recovery, they can be maintained with very palatable food, thus showing the importance of taste (Teitelbaum and Epstein 1962). Stress can also make them eat. This may be partly explained by damage done to dopamine-containing nigro striatal fibers.

In another classic experiment Hoebel (1979) demonstrated that obesity or hyperphagia in animals was induced by ventromedial lesions of the hypothalamus. Rats with medial hypothalamic lesions showed increased gastric secretion, hyperinsulinemia, and a hyperfunction of the parasympathetic system.

Though it seems much more understandable to analyze and discuss the functional states which have to do with eating behavior rather than anatomic structures and their lesions, we are primarily concerned with the structural background of hypothalamic nuclei and the amygdala (Powley 1977).

The diencephalic and limbic structures are probably the most important bases for transducing and integrating information from the external environment through the sensory apparatus, with one result being the emotional state. Metabolic input concerning the nutritional status of these structures will also be a factor in sense, control, and stabilization. These structures are rich in biologically active substances such as neurotransmitters and neurohormones, and therefore seem quite adapted to mediate monoamine and neuropeptide effects on food intake. These functions are embedded in various levels of brain network functions and interact with central and peripheral endocrine and autonomic processes.

The neurotransmitters taking part in the sensing and control of food intake, appetite, and energy control are the monoamines, namely NE, E, dopamine and serotonin. The amino acid gamma-aminobutyric acid is involved as well as a variety of neuropeptides, such as the pancreatic polypeptides, opioid peptides and hormone-releasing factors. Of these, neuropeptide Y has been shown to be one of the most potent stimulators of feeding (Stanley and Leibowitz 1984). Although it exists at various sites together with catecholamines, its action is independent of them. Neuropeptide Y, stemming from the family of pancreatic polypeptides, was isolated only in 1982. Its concentration in the brain is greater than that of any other putative neurotransmitter.

Other peptides have been reported to inhibit feeding. It was found that various peptides in different animal strains and at various sites may act either by increasing or decreasing food intake (especially the so-called satiety peptides), leaving the question open whether one is dealing with a satiety or a disruptive effect. In any case, most do act as such, thereby decreasing food intake. So far, these peptides have been identified as insulin, CCK, calcitonin, bombesin, neurotensin, somatostatin, TRH, CRF, and glucagon.

CCK most probably causes satiety through the inhibition of gastric emptying and consequent gastric distention. This effect seems to be relayed to the brain by afferent vagal fibers. L-phenylalanine, a releaser of CCK, produces reduction in food intake.

Neurotransmitter effects on eating behavior and potentially mediating brain areas will be shown schematically.

The Various Classes of Neurotransmitters

Eating-Stimulatory Neurotransmitters

Norepinephrine (NE) acts specifically to potentiate ingestion of carbohydrates, as opposed to proteins or fats. It also increases the size of the meal ingested and the rate of ingestion, rather than the frequency of meals taken. NE is important in the maintenance of feeding behavior.

The link between hypothalamic NE and carbohydrate ingestion can be related to the fact that NE, in order to function in this context, acts in close association with corticosterone and insulin, which of course have an important impact on carbohydrate metabolism (Shor-Posner et al. 1985). It has been demonstrated (Leibowitz et al. 1984; Leibowitz 1980) that the loss of response to NE subsequent to hypophysectomy is due to a disruption of the hypothalamic-pituitary-adrenal axis. The glucocorticoids of the adrenal gland appear to be the essential humoral factors interacting with paraventricular nucleus (PVN)-injected NE to elicit feeding.

Opioid peptides may mediate eating in cases of food deprivation or under conditions of painful stimulation and stress. Opioid peptides act also as analgesics and may work both in conjunction with or independently of NE. *Neuropeptide Y* and *peptide YYY* (Stanley and Leibowitz 1984) have a stimulatory effect on food intake. *GABA* (Kimura and Kuriyama 1975) has been found to act in a specific intermediary capacity in the link between glucose metabolism and central neural systems that control behavior.

Eating-Inhibitory Neurotransmitters

Serotonin exerts an inhibitory effect of feeding. It reduces the proportion of carbohydrate intake. In contrast, *hypothalamic dopamine receptors* may regulate appetite specifically for protein. *Fenfluoramine* has an anorectic effect, acting in part through the activation of serotonin. *Amphetamine,* by releasing brain catecholamines, may in part suppress feeding behavior through the inhibition of hunger processes which control meal initiation. Protein ingestion decreases brain uptake and consequently decreases serotonin synthesis. The serotonin system, in contrast, may control the process of meal termination through the activation of satiety mechanisms.

Monoamines in the hypothalamus are involved in the control of food intake and have specific effects on temporal feeding patterns as well as on appetite for specific food. Monoamines possibly take part in the satiety mechanism for carbohydrates, rather than in a hunger-stimulating process, with NE inhibiting and serotonin potentiating satiety, as might be expected.

There is also evidence that the macronutrients selected by a normal animal to satisfy its needs may themselves influence brain mechanisms that regulate food intake. Ingestion of food has been shown to alter plasma amino acid patterns, which in turn influence the entry of tyrosine and tryptophan into the brain, thus affecting the synthesis of catecholamines and serotonin. Similar links exist in relation to cortisone. Consumption of a carbohydrate meal at the beginning of the night results in a release of insulin and an increase in the concentration of plasma tryptophan relative to other neutral amino acids, which leads to an increase in the level of brain tryptophan and serotonin.

Brain peptides and monoamines coexist in a single neuron and may affect each other's pattern of release and receptor activity. Leibowitz (1985) and Morley et al. (1985) have suggested that these substances may interact closely in their control of appetite for food. Leibowitz and Shor-Posner (1986) arrived at a working hypothesis of hypothalamic monoamine functioning after having been deeply involved in this research for years. Leibowitz states:

> It is proposed that under decreased energy availability (e.g. at the start of the active period), an increase occurs in medial hypothalamic (PVN) alpha-2-noradrenergic activity, in association with a decline in 5-HT turnover and a rise in circulating CORT and insulin. Simultaneously, an increase in catecholaminergic activity in the perifornical lateral hypothalamus may also occur. Together, these transmitter changes, through effects respectively on satiety and hunger mechanisms, are expected to result in potentiated carbohydrate feeding, along with a simultaneous inhibition of protein ingestion. Since brain 5-HT synthesis, relative to CA synthesis, is increased after carbohydrate ingestion, a subsequent switch in preference for protein then occurs as a consequence of increased satiety for carbohydrate. With protein ingestion, the neurochemical profile then, shifts, once again, to an increase in hypothalamic CA synthesis and a decrease in 5-HT synthesis, followed by an enhanced preference for carbohydrate.
>
> Hypothalamic monoamines may also become activated in an unstable environment, such as when food is scarce and unpredictable or when the organism is stressed.

The Human Aspect

Leibowitz and Shor-Posner (1986) have also noted that bulimia could be primarily the result of increased medial hypothalamic alpha-noradrenergic activity, decreased medial hypothalamic serotonergic activity, or increased lateral hypothalamic dopaminergic or beta-adrenergic activity. It has been suggested that certain anorectic symptoms may at least in part be understood as a pathologic sympathetic neural function. Lateral hypothalamus stimulation, in contrast to lesions, causes eating responses. However, the lateral hypothalamus is also a reward (or pleasure) center, so that electrodes stimulating eating will also cause a pleasure effect. It is important to note that CCK, which is involved in satiety, has its receptors in the brain and spleen (the latter being considered as the brain of the immune system). The rich innervation of the gut with neuropeptides and neuropeptide receptors, and their involvement with pain and other sensations, immediately calls to mind the saying "gut feeling."

During bulimia, symptoms may be reversed by a sudden increase in alpha-noradrenergic activation, perhaps caused by the stress of drug administration. However, it is not simply an overcompensation of one system for another. As with many other functions, there are reciprocal interactions which stabilize the necessary equilibrium. On the other hand, extreme switches and sudden changes can be understood by the abrupt upset of this interaction of systems.

Thus, in the anorectic state, alpha-noradrenergic activity may be *depressed* through active inhibition from medial hypothalamic, serotonergic fiber systems, or from lateral hypothalamic, dopaminergic fiber systems. In contrast, in the bulimic state, symptoms of extreme noradrenergic activation (peripherally as well as in the medial hypothalamus) may be a consequence of attenuated serotonergic or dopaminergic function (Beaumont et al. 1976).

Other studies (Ball 1974; Sawchenko et al. 1981) have shown that the vagus nerve seems to be an important link through which neurohormones work. Halperin et al. (1983) showed that both electrical and adrenergic brain stimulation can induce eating in already satiated animals. In addition, he found that sub-diaphragmatic vagotomy abolishes eating elicited by both NE and electrical brain stimulation. Another interesting observation has been made by Flood et al. (1987) concerning memory-processing by CCK. This study investigated the memory function of animals concerning food availability, and found that CCK enhanced memory in mice. Furthermore, vagotomy interrupted this memory function. Here, ascending vagal fibers seemed to be the transmitters. This indicates that another link may have been found between the release of gastric peptides and memory-processing in the CNS, in this case because of the survival advantage of remembering the details of a successful food-foraging expedition.

In considering water homeostasis in anorectics, one should note that, at least in some animals, brain NE appears to play a part in control of vasopressin secretion. In the CSF and plasma of anorectics Gold et al. (1983) showed an increase in CSF vasopressin and in CSF/plasma vasopressin secretion rate, in addition to a disturbed pattern of vasopressin release in response to hypertonic saline.

Various experiments and hypotheses (i.e., Jhanwar-Uniyal et al. 1986) have shown that levels of neurotransmitters, enzymes, peptides, and metabolites fluctuate in the course of diurnal cycles. Such neurotransmitter changes participate in the regulation, control and rhythmicity of body temperature, release of anterior pituitary hormones, feeding, and drinking.

These experiments immediately suggest the possibility of medical drug treatment to correct the various increased or decreased monoamine functional states. However, up to now, no success has been achieved using drug treatment. The reasons for this lack of success are manifold. Firstly, this disequilibrium is not a simple over- or under-functioning of one system or another. It is rather an interplay of many factors with possibly reciprocal inhibitory and/or disinhibitory effects. Secondly, we are not able to foresee or predict the different functions of the various amines and peptides at their sites of action. It is therefore difficult to introduce drugs into those systems and to control their complex mechanisms. And finally, the psychological make-up of the patient, one of a motivational state to fight and control ingestion, makes it extremely difficult to use drugs effectively. In cases where hunger was increased in anorectic patients, their response was to control this feeling even more and to refuse all medication. Indeed, it is our clinical experience that when trying to influence noradrenergic or dopaminergic activity by introducing appetite stimuli the result was the end of any kind of positive therapeutic relationship.

We have tried to demonstrate the present state of knowledge concerning neurotransmitter function in relation to food intake. The complexity of these findings is heightened by the fact that these functional states vacillate continuously, which means that equilibrium is relative to certain internal "needs" and states. These discoveries, some of which are not synchronous with psychological findings, make it extremely difficult to correlate physiological and psychological elements.

Endocrine Functioning

Cortisol

At one time it was hypothesized that anorexia nervosa was a form of adrenal insufficiency, but this turned out to be untrue. It was subsequently shown that the adrenal cortex of anorectics was more responsive than normal. These patients responded to the administration of adrenocorticotropic hormone (ACTH) by exaggerated cortisol response. Thus, in the anorectic, the hypothalamic-pituitary-adrenal axis is possibly even more active than usual. Morning and evening levels of cortisol are usually higher than in healthy subjects, as is also true of the 24 h mean plasma cortisol concentrations. The high levels of basal plasma cortisol are possibly due to alterations in binding globulin with a circadian rhythm that is flattened at higher levels, an increased production rate (stress), a decreased metabolic clearance rate, and a prolonged half-life of the hormone.

Growth hormone production in anorectics is generally increased, though it normalizes with recovery. This phenomenon is linked with specific caloric intake. Often the growth hormone response to a glucose load is a paradoxical increase. The response to insulin stimulation is usually blunted.

Thyroid Function

The function of the pituitary-thyroid axis of anorectics is impaired, with low basal levels of triiodothyronine (T_3). Thyroxine (T_4), however, was reported to be normal. Thyroid-stimulating hormone (TSH) levels were mostly normal to high with a delayed response to TRH stimulation. These phenomena seem to be related to the starvation syndrome in general, especially to carbohydrate deficiency. Palmblad et al. (1977) have shown this hypothyroid-like syndrome in starving human beings, with reduced metabolic rate, hypothermia, dry skin, elevated serum cholesterol, and bradycardia. In general, as stated by Fichter and Pirke (1986), disturbances in the hypothalamic-pituitary-thyroid axis (as well as other neuroendorince axes) are secondary to a reduced caloric intake and a catabolic state.

The impairment which underlies *amenorrhea* is a result of the plasma and urinary levels of two pituitary polypeptides, luteinizing hormone (LH) and follicle-stimulating hormone (FSH), being low during the active phase of anorexia nervosa. Katz et al. (1977) assume that this is the result of the LH and FSH synthesized by the pituitary not being released in normal fashion because the hypothalamic mechanism that controls their release by the pituitary is defective. A linear relationship has also been found between resting levels of plasma LH and body weight. LH levels are normalized as weight is regained. In addition, baseline FSH values are reduced and return to normal with weight gain.

Interestingly, Garfinkel et al. (1981) have shown that anorectic patients with weight loss have 24 h secretory patterns of serum gonadotropins resembling those in normal prepubertal or pubertal girls. Donovan (1965) had demonstrated that in recovery from anorexia nervosa hypothalamic-pituitary-gonadal activity returns in a definite sequence that recapitulates puberty. In both animals and humans, studies on the function of gonadal steroid hormones (Kakolewski et al. 1982; Wade and Zucker 1970) found that they influence food intake. Food intake of the estrous rat varies inversely with the plasma estradiol concentration, suggesting that estradiol has an inhibitory effect on food intake. Removal of the endogenous source of estrogens by ovariectomy results in a sharp rise in food intake and gain in body weight.

Fishman (1975) studied the metabolism of tracer estradiol in young women with anroexia nervosa and compared it to normal and obese controls. He found that the malnourished females converted estradiol to 2-hydroxyestrone to a far greater extent than the other controls. He later showed that in animals hypophagia was caused by excessive amounts of 2-hydroxyestrone. The role of progesterone and testosterone in food intake is less well defined.

The cause of early amenorrhea is controversial. Menstrual disturbances often antedate other obvious manifestations by several months. Many researchers (e.g., Russell 1972) believe that amenorrhea is caused by unspecific stress factors (as seen in wartime or during internment) as well as changes in climatic conditions. Rose et al. (1983) also believe that it can be initiated by stress. An increased secretion of adrenal corticosteroids and catecholamines affects the hypothalamic control of gonadotropins. In contrast, Guevara et al. (1970) doubted if gonadotropins were stress-dependent hormones, although believed that ACTH, growth hormone, and prolactin were stress dependent. Meyer et al. (1986) recently compared amenorrhea and predictors for "remenorrhea" in anorectic patients. He found that early (preceding weight loss) amenorrhea was associated with less anorexia-specific psychological traits and more weight loss later.

As is well known, athletic women and ballet dancers often have amenorrhea and seem undernourished. Malina et al. (1978) suggested that there may be a selection factor at work that induces women with partially poor menstrual functions to opt for strenuous exercise.

From the cited material it can be seen that most, if not all, endocrine deviant findings can be explained by metabolic adaptation to reduced caloric intake. Changes in the pituitary-adrenal axis can be conditioned by changed cortisol mechanisms induced by the decrease of T_3. Impaired thermoregulation, hypotension, and bradycardia are probably related to decreased sympathetic activity.

To summarize, it is still very difficult to state whether anorectics suffer from only some functional disturbance of the hypothalamus, or if there is more than a secondary involvement of the hypothalamic-pituitary-adrenal axis. This question can only be resolved through the investigation of dynamic patterns of endocrine functions. In any case, because of the interwoven nature of emotional and endocrine functioning, it is only possible to discuss the nature and character of anorexia as a real psychosomatic disorder.

Trace Elements

Low dietary intake has many consequences which are essentially connected with low energy supply, storage, and reuse. Vitamin supply is usually sufficient in anorectics since a common family reaction is to provide them with vitamin supplements in pill form, which are usually taken without hesitation. However, many vitamin supplements do not contain essential minerals. Numerous minerals and trace metals are used by the body in various enzymatic processes. It it therefore important in anorectics to check mineral levels which may be deficient as a result of their low food intake.

The possible connection between deficient levels of trace metals and anorexia nervosa has pointed to two basic directions of study: (a) the possibility of a primary disorder of trace metal uptake and deviation in resorption, and (b) whether mineral metabolism could be disturbed due to damage to the intestinal mucosa. Underwood (1978) reviewed the influence of low intake of dietary protein and energy upon the intake and physiologic availability and utilization of trace elements. He found that kwashiorkor, an illness which produces emaciation, is also noted for a deficiency of chromium. It was also found that cow's milk, as compared with human milk, is relatively poor in copper and infants who are nourished solely on cow's milk may therefore suffer from copper deficiency. Some infant formulae have also been shown to be deficient in zinc, especially soy-protein-based formulae rather than milk-protein-based formulae. Zinc deficiency is usually associated with low protein diets.

Various studies (Hansen et al. 1983; Gordon et al. 1981; Oelshigel and Brewer 1977) have further shown that some copper and zinc aberrations are connected with certain CNS diseases. It has been conjectured that zinc deficiency, found in some cases of anorexia nervosa, may have some contributory etiologic value. This conjecture stemmed from the fact that some symptoms of anorexia are similar to those of primary zinc deficiency, namely, dryness of the skin, loss of hair, anemia, and increased plasma carotene levels. However, it has proved impossible to localize any of these dysfunctions since zinc is essential for the functioning of more than 50 metabolic enzymes.

It is known that trace metals compete with each other in biologic systems. An excess of copper in tissues can block access to an active enzyme site by a more effective metal such as zinc. Copper is said to be a CNS stimulant, while zinc is a sedative. Casper et al. (1980) have worked extensively on serum zinc levels in female patients with anorexia nervosa. They showed that these patients had distorted taste and smell, alopecia, hypogonadism, and an elevated pain threshold – all signs of zinc deficiency. They also found, together with the zinc deficiency, high vitamin A and carotene levels. It should be noted that other disturbances were found in zinc-deficient organisms, such as poor wound-healing and increased sensitivity to insulin. Vitamin A cannot be utilized by the body unless adequate amounts of zinc are present. Zinc has been implicated in the synthesis of retinol-binding protein (RBP), a protein necessary for vitamin A transport from the liver to other organs.

It is important to remember that zinc deficiency is relative, being dependent on metabolic requirements. In all likelihood, the low metabolic rate of anorectic patients reduces tissue requirements for zinc. Casper illustrated this by finding normal zinc content in the hair of anorectic patients. From this, she concluded that the abnormalities in the levels of micronutrients in the blood of anorectic patients were either directly or indirectly related to nutrition.

Another interesting interpretation explaining the postprandial low serum zinc concentration in anorexia nervosa was given by Dinsmore et al. (1985).

They found that anorectics had reduced zinc absorption, which under normal conditions could result in impaired small-intestinal metabolism, and thus a self-perpetuating state could be created in which food restriction leads to lower zinc intake with impaired cellular function and clinical anorexia, which in turn leads to dietary restriction and further zinc deficiency.

Bryce-Smith and Simpson (1984) showed that not only starvation but also other stresses increased urinary zinc excretion, thereby exacerbating the effect of reduced dietary intake. They also reported a case of an anorectic girl being cured with zinc sulphate. Akar (1984) suggested another link between zinc deficiency and anorexia nervosa: oestrogens enhance the excretion of zinc, so that there is increased risk of zinc deficiency in young females, especially if they use oral contraceptives. The zinc deficiency may be a factor in producing amenorrhea and may even be exacerbated by the use of oral contraceptives which are often prescribed to treat amenorrhea. This may be true especially in those anorectic patients in which amenorrhea precedes the onset of weight loss.

In an unpublished report from 1987, M. Statter, Z. Schumert, E. Moguilner, and E. L. Edelstein examined zinc status and serum prolactin concentrations in 10 patients with anorexia nervosa using zinc loading tests. Two groups of patients could be distinguished, one with normal fasting plasma levels (82.0 ± 10.0 ug/dl) and normal zinc tolerance tests, and one with decreased plasma zinc levels (65 ± 9.1 μg/dl. M ± SD; *P* 0.01) and low plasma zinc concentrations following the test (50 mg of elemental zinc ingested). It is interesting to note that the first group of patients had been suffering from anorexia for less than 5 years, while the latter group had had it for a longer period of time. Basal prolactin levels were found to be normal in all the anorectic patients, and zinc ingestion appeared to have no influence on prolactin concentration in the serum.

Although these above-mentioned findings do not provide convincing etiologic evidence for anorexia nervosa, it is important to point out the very interesting results of an immunologic study involving zinc by Fraker et al. (1986). They demonstrated the importance of zinc to host defense and immune ontogeny. Zinc was shown to be the element best able to influence immune functions. Nevertheless, in relation to anorectic symptoms, it must be concluded that zinc, other trace metals, and various biochemical elements are diminished in quantity with the decreased need and metabolism of an emaciated body.

Organic Brain Elements

EEG Patterns

Although in general there has been little research done concerning EEG patterns or brain pathology in anorectics, there have been some interesting, if unspecific findings. EEG patterns are neglected at present due to the development of better techniques of brain research such as computerized tomograpy (CT) scans, magnetic resonance techniques, and positron emission tomography (PET). EEG findings such as "paroxysmal slowing", "mitten patterns", "minimal generalized slow", "minimal generalized fast", "small sharp spikes", and others are designated unspecific as related to well-defined diseases.

Nevertheless, some interest has been devoted to the "14 and 6 per second positive spike" syndrome and its connection to certain episodic autonomous behavior disturbances. Low success rates were reported with phenytoin treatment in this syndrome, both in the EEG and in behavior. For example, Gibbs and Gibbs (1951) found a relatively high incidence (21%) of 14 and 6 per second positive spike pattern among unselected children and adolescents. Demerdash et al. (1968) found an incidence of 14.2% in unselected youngsters, while Gianturco et al. (1972) found a high incidence (56%) of positive spike pattern in patients who had both psychiatric disorders and autonomic complaints (paroxysmal character) when compared to patients with only a psychiatric disorder (19%) and patients with only autonomic complaints (29%).

Studying these patterns in nutritional disorders, Shimoda and Kitagawa (1973) examined 14 and 6 per second positive spikes and 6 per second spikes and wave activity (phantoms) as well as "mitten patterns." They found 14 and 6 per second positive spike patterns especially in abstaining anorectics, as well as in bulimics and binge eaters. Rau et al. (1979) examined the EEG of 59 compulsive eaters and found an abnormality rate of 64.4%, which is much higher than in normal controls. If one relates binge eating to a lack of self-control, the ensuing dysrhythmia is understandable; 71.1% of the abnormal EEGs displayed either 14 and 6 per second positive spikes or the B-mitten pattern. From this evidence Rau et al. assumed that both patterns presented evidence of subcortical origin.

In contrast, Maulsby (1979) claimed that the 14 and 6 per second positive spikes are not specific and may occur in adolescents with other complaints. Nevertheless, the fact remains that some good therapeutic results were obtained with phenytoin treatment; for example, Rau and Green (1975) found that it helped not only psychiatric and autonomous symptoms, but also episodic aggressive behavior, temper tantrums, irritability, and insomnia, as well as compulsive, uncontrollable attacks of stealing or cleaning.

In eating disorders, Green and Rau (1977) reported success with diphenylhydantoin (DPH) treatment in nine out of ten bulimic patients. In a more controlled study with a double-blind cross-over design, Wermuth et al. (1977) achieved a more moderate but still impressive and statistically significant reduction in binge eating by phenytoin administration. Rau et al. (1979) showed that 70% of patients with abnormal EEGs improved with DPH, as compared with only a 35.3% improvement rate for those bingers with normal EEGs. The improvement rate of these compulsive eaters with 14 and 6 per second positive spikes, following DPH treatment, was 88.9%, which was substantially higher than the improvement rate for other EEG abnormalities. Furthermore, Rau showed that when underweight and overweight patients with nutritional disorders (called "deviant weight" group) were combined, 15 of the 18 patients with abnormal EEGs responded well to DPH as compared with only two of the seven patients with normal EEGs. This association is highly significant statistically ($P = 0.0003$).

In our own work we treated four anorectics who had some form of unspecific EEG disturbance with DPH. This treatment was used because all four of these patients exhibited several forms of paroxysmal uncontrolled behavior. One patient had attacks of binge eating or bulimia. The other three exhibited temper tantrums and aggressive, mostly autoaggressive, behavior which occurred in unexpected attacks. When given DPH in adequate doses all four patients' behavior improved, and neither they themselves nor their parents complained of any further attacks. When this medication was withdrawn after a period of a few weeks the impulsive attacks of uncontrollable character returned, to disappear again when the drug was readministered.

Hughes, one of the major skeptics concerning the use of DPH, conducted further experiments on the 14 and 6 per second positive spike syndrome, to see if it should be considered a normal variant or as a sign of pathology (Hughes and Cayaffa 1978). He was particularly interested in finding out whether the specific EEGs would continue in an adult population. He designed a well-controlled study which involved 460 adults who were found to have the 14 and 6 per second positive spike pattern", out of a total sample population of 50000 people. Hughes found that females had the syndrome more often, in a male/female ratio of 32:68. Neurovegetative (61%) or psychiatric (41%) complaints were more often found in 85% of the adults with this wave form. It is interesting to note that the incidence of neurovegetative complaints was greater here than in all comparison groups except those with normal EEGs. Neil et al. (1980) found that 34.5% of anorectics display some sort of abnormal "slow background activity." This was seen as possibly reflecting some endocrine changes.

It is our hypothesis that in all the dyscontrol syndromes there is some uncontrollable, dysrhythmic, and impulsive element of behavior. This type of cyclical behavior is most often termed regressive, and relates to both psychic and organic regression. Regression of this type can be seen as similar to "impulsive behavior." It is therefore interesting to note that the more uncontrolled a certain behavior may be, as in temper tantrums or bulimic and episodic eating attacks, the more an anticonvulsive drug – which works on some brain immaturity or subcortical cerebral dysrhythmia – will be successful. This is a further illustration of how certain somatopsychic elements correspond with brain mechanisms. It also seems to suggest an increased serotonergic function and possibly decreased adrenergic activity which enhances the effectiveness of the drug.

Brain Atrophy

Besides the biochemical and endocrine changes which occur in the brain after fasting, certain physical changes take place as well. Kohlmeyer et al. (1983); Enzmann and Lane (1977); Nussbaum et al. (1980); Sein et al. (1981) all found that malnutrition leads to severe protein loss and fluid retention in the brain, which may be a pathophysiological base for brain atrophy or so-called pseudoatrophy of the brain. Kohlmeyer, using computed tomography in patients with anorexia nervosa (Kohlmeyer et al. 1983), found pronounced symmetrical enlargement of cortical sulci. Enlargement of the subarachnoid space was indicated by the prominence of the insular cisterns and the anterior interhemispheric fissure. Both Kohlmeyer and other researchers could not explain these changes, except as the possible result of protein deficiency. Surprisingly, with the attainment of normal weight the cerebral atrophy disappeared. It is for this reason that researchers in this field speak of the syndrome of reversibility of atrophy or of a pseudoatrophy of the brain.

Further progress in measuring the physiological state of anorectic patients has been achieved by the use of positron emission tomography (PET). Emrich et al. (1984) found that in contrast to the pronounced cortical pseudoatrophy, the cortical glucose metabolism of anorectic patients seems to be normal (as demonstrated by PET scan). This could be an important step in the measurement of functional states.

References

Akar N (1984) Anorexia and zinc, letter to the editor. Lancet II: 874

Ball CG (1974) Vagotomy: effect on electrically induced eatings and self stimulation in the lateral hypothalamus. Science 184: 484–485

Ban T (1966) The septo-preoptico-hypothalamic system and its automatic function. In: Tokizane T, Schacte JP (eds) Progress in brain research, vol 21A. Elsevier, Amsterdam, pp 1–43

Beaumont PJV, George GCW, Pimstone BL, Vinik AI (1976) Body weight and the pituitary response to hypothalamic releasing hormones in patients with anorexia nervosa. J Clin Endocrinol 43: 487

Bray GA, York DA (1979) Hypothalamic and genetic obesity in experimental animals: an automatic and endocrine hypothesis. Physiol Rev 59: 719–808

Bryce-Smith D, Simpson RID (1984) Letter to the editor. Lancet 2: 874

Casper RC, Kirschner B, Sandstead HH, Jacob RA, Davis JM (1980) An evaluation of trace metals, vitamins and taste function in anorexia nervosa. Am J Clin Nutr 33: 1801–1808

Crisp AH, Ellis J, Lowy C (1967) Insulin response to a rapid intravenous injection of dextrose in patients with anorexia nervosa and obesity. Postgrad Med 43: 97–102

Demerdash A, Olofason O, Peterson I (1968) The incidence of 14 and 6 per second positive spikes in a population of normal children. Dev Med Child Neurol 10: 309–316

Dinsmore WW, Alderdice JT, McMaster D, Adams CEA, Love AHG (1985) Zinc absorption in anorexia nervosa, letter to the editor. Lancet 1: 1041–1042

Donovan BT (1965) Der werfften bosch. J.J. Physiology of puberty. Monographs of the Physiological Society. Arnold, London

Emrich HM, Pahl JJ, Herholz K, Pavlik G, Pirka KM, Gerlinghoff M, Wienhard W, Heiss WD (1984) PET investigation in anorexia nervosa: normal glucose metabolism during pseudo-atrophy of the brain. In: Pirke KM, Ploog D (eds) The psychobiology of anorexia nervosa. Springer, Berlin Heidelberg New York

Enzmann DR, Lane B (1977) Cranial computed tomography findings in anorexia nervosa. J Comput Assist Tomogr 1:410–414

Fichter MM, Pirke KM (1986) Effects of experimental starvation on the thyroid axis. In: Brambilla FE (ed) Disorders of eating behavior: a psychoendocrine approach: advances of the biosciences. Pergamon, Oxford, pp 189–198

Fishman J (1975) Appetite and sex hormone. In: Silverston T (ed) Dahlem workshop on appetite and food intake 2(7):218

Flood JF, Smith GE, Morley JE (1987) Modulation of memory processing by cholecystokinin: dependence on the vagus nerve. Science 236:832–834

Fraker PG, Gershwin ME, Good RA, Prasad A (1986) Interrelationships between zinc and immune function. Fed Proc 45:1474–1479

Garfinkel PE, Brown GM, Darby PL (1981) The psychoendocrinology of anorexia nervosa. Int J Ment Health 9:162–193

Gianturco DT, Wilson WP, Mursella L (1972) Effect of psychiatric and autonomous symptoms on the incidence of fourteen and six per second positive spikes among adolescents. Clin Electroencephalography 3(1):55–59

Gibbs EL, Gibbs EA (1951) Electroencephalographic evidence of thalamic and hypothalamic epilepsy. Neurology 1:136–144

Gold PW, Kaye W, Robertson GL, Ebert M (1983) Abnormalities in plasma and cerebrospinal fluid arginine vasopressin in patients with anorexia nervosa. N Engl J Med 308:1117–1123

Gordon E, Gordon RC, Passal DB (1981) Zinc metabolism, basic, clinical and behavioral aspects. J Pediatr 99:341–349

Green RS, Rau JH (1977) The use of diphenylhydantoin in compulsive eating disorders. In: Vigersky RA (ed) Anorexia nervosa. Raven, New York, pp 377–382

Grossman SP (1975) Role of the hypothalamus in the regulation of food and water intake. Psychol Rev 82:200–224

Guevara A, Luria MH, Wieland RE (1970) Serum gonadotrophin level during medical stress. Metabolism 19:79–83

Halmi KA (1978) Anorexia nervosa: recent investigations. Annu Rev Med 29:137–148

Halperin R, Gatchalian CL, Adachi TJ, Carter J, Leibowitz SF (1983) Relationship of adrenergic and electrical brain stimulation induced feeding response. Pharmacol Biochem Behav 18:415–422

Hansen CR, Malecha M, Mackenzie TB, Kroll J (1983) Copper and zinc deficiencies in association with depression and neurological findings. Biol Psychiatry 18(3):395–401

Hoebel BG (1979) Hypothalamic self-stimulation and stimulation escape in relation to feeding and mating. Fed Proc 38:2454–2461

Hughes JR, Cayaffa JJ (1978) Positive spikes revisited in the adult. Clin Electroencephalography 9(2):52–59

Jhanwar-Uniyal M, Roland CR, Leibowitz SF (1986) Diurnal rhythm of alpha-2 noradrenergic receptors in the paraventricular nucleus and other brain areas: relation to circulating corticosterone and feeding behavior. Life Sci 38:473–482

Kakolewski JW, Cox VC, Valenstein ES (1982) Sex differences in body weight change following gonadectomy of rats. Psychol Rep 22:547–554

Katz JL, Boyar RM, Weiner H, Gorzynski G, Roffwarg H, Hellman L (1976) Toward an elucidation of the psychoneuroendocrinology of anorexia nervosa. In: Sachar E (ed) Hormones, behavior and psychopathology. Raven, New York, pp 263–283

Katz JL, Boyar R, Roffwarg H, Hellman L, Weiner H (1977) LHRH responsiveness in anorexia nervosa: intactness despite prepubertal circadian LH pattern. Psychosom Med 39:4

Katz JL, Boyar R, Roffwarg H, Hellman L, Weiner H (1978) Weight and circadian luteinizing hormone secretory pattern in anorexia nervosa. Psychosom Med 40:549–567

Kaye WH, Ebert MH, Lake CR (1980) Central nervous system amine metabolism in anorexia nervosa. The 133 annual meeting of the American Psychiatric Association syllabus and scientific Proceedings, p 326

Kimura H, Kuriyama K (1975) Distribution of gamma-aminobutyric acid in the rat hypothalamus: Functional correlates of GABA with activities of appetite-controlling mechanisms. J Neurochem 24:903–907

Kohlmeyer K, Lehmkuhl G, Poustka F (1983) Computed tomography in patients with anorexia nervosa. AJNR 4:437–438

Leibowitz SF (1980) Neurochemical systems of the hypothalamus: control of feeding and drinking behavior and water-electrolyte excretion. In: Morgane PJ, Panksepp J (eds) Handbook of the hypothalamus, vol 34. Dekker, New York, pp 299–437

Leibowitz SF (1985) Brain neurotransmitters and appetite regulation. Psychopharmacol Bull 21:418–421

Leibowitz SF, Shor-Posner G (1986) Hypothalamic monoamine systems for control of food intake: analysis of meal pattern and macro-nutrient selection. In: Corruber MO, Blundell JE (eds) Pharmacology of eating disorders: theoretical and clinical developments. Raven, New York

Leibowitz SF, Roland CR, Hor L, Squillari V (1984) Noradrenergic feeding elicited via the paraventricular nucleus is dependent upon circulating corticosterone. Physiol Behav 32:857–864

Malina RM, Spirduso WW, Tate C, Baylor AM (1978) Age at menarche and selected menstrual characteristics in athletes. Med Sci Sports 10:218–222

Maulsby RL (1979) EEG patterns of uncertain diagnostic significance. In: Klass DQ, Daly DD (eds) Current practice of clinical electroencephalography. Raven, New York

Meyer AE, Von Holtzapfel B, Deffner G, Engle K, Klick M (1986) Amenorrhoea and predictors for remenorrhoea in anorexia nervosa: psychoendocrinological study in patients. Psychother Psychosom 45:149–160

Morley JE, Levine AS, Gosnell BA, Krahn DD (1985) Peptides as central regulators of feeding. Brain Res Bull 14:511–519

Neil JF, Merikanges JR, Foster FG, Merikanges KR, Spiker DG, Kupfer DJ (1980) Waking and all-night sleep EEGs in anorexia nervosa. Clin Electroencephalography 11:9–15

Nussbaum M, Shenker JR, Marc J, Klein M (1980) Cerebral atrophy in anorexia nervosa. J Pediatr 96:867–869

Oelshigel FJ, Brewer GJ (1977) Absorption of pharmacological doses of zinc. In: Brewer GJ, Prasa AS (eds) Zinc metabolism: current aspects in health and disease. Liss, New York, pp 299–311

Palmblad J, Levi L, Burger A, Melander A, Westgren U, Schlenk H von, Skusle K (1977) Effect of total energy withdrawal (fasting) on the levels of growth hormone, thyrotropin, cortisol, adrenaline, noradrenaline, T_4 and T_3 in healthy males. Acta Med Scand 201:15–22

Powley TL (1977) The ventromedial hypothalamic syndrome, satiety and a cephalic phase hypothesis. Psychol Rev 84:89–126

Rau JH, Green RS (1975) Compulsive eating: a neuropsychological approach to certain eating disorders. Compr Psychiatry 16(3):223–231

Rau JH, Struve FA, Green RS (1979) Electroencephalographic correlates of compulsive eating. Clin Electroencephalography 10(4):180–189

Rose E (1983) Fatness and reproduction: delayed menarche and amenorrhoea of ballet dancers and college athletes. In: Darby PL (ed) Anorexia nervosa: recent developments in research. Liss, New York, pp 343–363
Russell GFM (1972) Psychological and nutritional factors in disturbances of menstrual function and ovulation. Postgrad Med J 48:10–13
Sawchenko PE, Gold RM, Leibowitz SF (1981) Evidence for vagal involvement in eating elicited by adrenergic stimulation of the paraventricular nucleus. Brain Res 225:249–269
Sein P, Searson S, Nicol AR, Hall K (1981) Anorexia nervosa and pseudoatrophy of the brain. Br J Psychiatry 139:257–258
Shimoda Y, Kitagawa T (1973) Clinical and EEG studies on the emaciation (anorexia nervosa) due to disturbed function of the brain stem. J Neural Transm 34:195–204
Shor-Posner G, Grinker JA, Marinescu C, Leibowitz SF (1985) Role of hypothalamic norepinephrine in control of meal patterns. Physiol Behav 35:209–214
Stanley BG, Leibowitz SF (1984) Neuropeptide Y: stimulation of feeding and drinking by injection into the paraventricular nucleus. Life Sci 35:2635–2642
Teitelbaum P, Epstein AN (1962) The lateral hypothalamic syndrome: recovery of feeding and drinking after lateral hypothalamic lesions. Psychol Rev 69:74–90
Underwood EJ (1978) Changes in trace metals in protein or energy restriction. J Hum Nutr 32(4):253–257
Wade GN, Zucker I (1970) Development of hormonal control over food intake and body weight in female rats. J Comp Physiol Psychol 70:213–220
Wermuth BM, Davis KL, Hollister LE, Stunkard AJ (1977) Phenytoin treatment of the binge-eating syndrome. Am J Psychiatry 134:1249–1253

CHAPTER 6

Bulimia – A Subgroup of Anorexia or a Separate Disease?

"There is no love sincerer than the love of food."

G. B. Shaw, *Man and Superman*, 1, 1903

The question of whether bulimia can be classified as a separate disease or as a part of the anorexia nervosa syndrome is still unresolved. The approach taken to this question depends on both the aspects investigated and compared, as well as the school of thought of the therapist and the resulting conception of the development of the disease and its subsequent treatment.

Bulimia is the addictive side of the coin of eating disorders. It is characterized by pure impulse. In contrast, in anorexia, one can only assume the covert, implicit element of impulse. What is observable is only the reaction to the strength of the impulse, the compulsive overcontrol and masochistic behavior. It is in this respect, however, that both diseases exhibit severe fixation or regression to an early developmental phase, in which object relations are more or less of an autistic character. In both diseases the body is a part object, and food is personified as an object, though related to it in different ways.

Boskind-Lodahl et al. (1978) resolved the issue of the classification of bulimia by calling the syndrome "bulimarexia," thus showing that the disease contained characteristics of classical anorexia nervosa. Others called it "binge-purge syndrome." I myself tend towards the concept of bulimia being part of the spectrum of anorectic disorders. Anorexia and bulimia belong to the same category with regard to character formation, the extent of regression, and object relation. This conceptualization is similar to that of manic-depressive disease. Just as the manic phase and the depressive phase are actually extreme poles of the same disturbance, so too are anorexia and bulimia extreme poles of the same disorder. This is also true in the psychodynamic sense, in which both impotence and omnipotence are expressed in either the anorectic or bulimic phases. Bulimia can be seen as the direct expression of the impulse while anorexia is the expression of the oversuppression of the very same impulse.

This conceptualization is borne out by the fact that most anorectics, when not in treatment, at times exhibit episodes of bulimic behavior. After such an episode the anorectic practices some sort of purification ritual and then reenters an anorectic phase of behavior. It is interesting to note that when impulsive mechanisms like bulimic episodes prevail, they are shorter than the anorectic phase and show an "attack" form. These attacks are usually sudden, and this characteristic is also demonstrated by the various types of dysrhythmic or otherwise disturbed EEGs that some anorectics exhibit. Most of these individuals respond well to the administration of an anticonvulsive drug such as DPH, which also has an antiaggressive effect (probably via the pathways of the amygdala).

Many bulimics, though not fat, often have similar or identical delusional body images as anorectics (such as seeing their hips as too big, and having fantasies of cutting off perceived oversized parts of the body). I had a bulimic-anorectic patient who, though not thin, had to eat constantly. At the same time she took close to a hundred laxatives a day in order to "cleanse" her body, at which point she was then able to resume her eating experiences. This need to cleanse the body is essentially similar to the ascetic mechanism of anorectics. In contrast, however, the social element in bulimics is not so disturbed. The bulimic is not perceived as a real anorectic and, therefore, will not be as conspicuous and will be able to achieve superficial object relations.

The fear of being unable to stop eating is common to both anorexia and bulimia; it is the fear of inevitability, of going on and on, the fear of something one cannot break. This cycle is well demonstrated in some of Escher's artistic expression. There is probably a connection between this fear and that of orgastic feelings in some women.

Bulimic attacks also happen during certain phases of dynamic therapy, especially when patients cannot deal with inner anxiety or when therapy threatens them with the opening up of some aspect which requires the expression of deep emotions. Under these circumstances, food is used to enclose those emotions, by the act of devouring everything. It is, therefore, when overcontrol is broken down that compulsive eating, as well as rage and temper tantrums, result. Kleptomania in bulimics can be seen as a release of stored rage, the expression of excitement of impulses, and the need to relieve tension.

Casper (1980) tried to evaluate the characteristics of patients with bulimic attacks. He studied 105 patients who met the criteria for anorexia nervosa. Bulimia was found to be associated with a typical symptom pattern; bulimic patients manifested greater anxiety, depression, guilt, and interpersonal sensitivity, and had more somatic complaints. Casper also found that vomiting and kleptomania happened exclusively in the bulimics. She concluded that the more outgoing personality characteristics of bulimic patients, in connection with diminished impulse and self-control as apparent in a distinct psychiatric symptomatology, differentiate them from fasting patients into a subgrup of anorexia nervosa.

Pure bulimics (a concept somewhat similar to obesity) behave differently from bulimic-anorectic patients. Their behavior is obviously impulsive and their quality of object relation is somewhat more mature. Pure bulimics do have at least superficial object relations. This distinction is noted by Herzog and Copeland (1985) who stated that:

Anorexia nervosa is a syndrome characterized by extreme weight loss, body-image disturbance and an intense fear of becoming obese. Bulimia is a syndrome distinct from anorexia nervosa and is characterized by secretive binge eating episodes followed by self-induced vomiting, fasting or the use of laxatives or diuretics. Bulimic symptoms can also be a part of the anorexia nervosa syndrome. An intense preoccupation with food is common to both syndromes.

In conclusion, most clinicians dealing with nutritional disorders classify bulimia as a subgroup of anorexia nervosa, though it exhibits somewhat milder character deviances. Bulimia may occur in about half of anorexia cases as a phase of the illness, with or without treatment.

References

Boskind-Lodahl M, White WC (1978) The definition and treatment of bulminarexia in college women: a pilot study. J Am Coll Health 27 [2]: 84–86

Casper RC, Eckert ED, Halmi KA, Goldberg SC, Davis JM (1980) Bulimia, its incidence and clinical importance in patients with anorexia nervosa. Arch Gen Psychiatry 37: 1030–1035

Herzog DB, Copeland (1985) Eating disorders. N Engl J Med 313: 295–303

CHAPTER 7

Obesity

"To eat well is no whoredom; and to starve is not gentility."

Thoman Fuller: Gnomologie, 1732

In general, obesity is the outcome of a positive energy balance, in which the caloric intake is greater than the energy output. The reason why obese people overeat is the subject of much interest and concern in the medical profession. Schachter (1968) suggested that external (nonvisceral) cues, not visceral hunger stimulus, are the regulating factors for eating in obese people. These individuals seem to be unresponsive to physiological hunger signals such as gastric hypermotility and blood sugar levels. Schachter also showed that obese people are hyperresponsive to cognitive and sensory qualities of food. In contrast, both Kincey (1981) and Isbitzki and Romano White (1981) had difficulty in verifying these findings. From these results and others, a controversy exists on the exact causes of overeating.

In spite of this controversy it seems clear that, if no hormonal aberration is demonstrated, the obese are more responsive to external cues, are more arousable in general, and may also be motivated to eat by the abundance and palatability of supermarket products. A similar process may exist in the abuse of drugs, in which availability is an element of seductive value.

Examples of Rationalizations for Overeating

"Eating is a common social experience" (this sounds simple and rational).
"I am eating well-earned food, which I deserve after a difficult experience."
"Food is the only pleasure in life; Let me enjoy it" (orality).
"I have earned food through my behavior" (eating in a festive mood) – "it was such a satisfying day!".

Food is also used when bored or when in a depressive mood to try to fill oneself concretely. Eating out of inner tension, in order to fill and soothe, is also used. Food can fill the need to have something in the mouth which may be part of the aggressive element of fantasizing about the power to devour cannibalistically. Eating is also used in order to hoard food within the body. It is an expression of the fear of not having enough later, a mechanism of insurance in time of continuity. Food can also be used to produce the excitement of being in transition to altered states of awareness, and as with other addictions it can be used to deny reality and to produce numbness and apathy toward the world within and without.

When examining the problem of overeating it is important to take into account developmental factors, or rather developmental deficits. It can be assumed that at a certain infantile stage unpleasantness was amorphic and diffuse. Dissatisfaction or displeasure were not yet differentiated into hunger, fear, pain, and anger. The obese seem to have not learned to differentiate between sensations and emotions. Therefore any state of arousal may be sensed as hunger, which is the earliest satisfying mechanism, the bodily reaction leading most quickly and concretely to satisfaction and pleasure.

For the more developed personality, overeating may be a defense against loneliness, depression, and anxiety. It can also be used in a more negative way, as a means of expressing shame, self-contempt, and self-rejection. Some individuals may eat in a compulsive way to suppress their ambivalence. There seems to be much truth in the old clinical saying that fat, having an insulation quality, is used for a defensive function.

References

Isbitzki JR, Romano White D (1981) Externality and locus of control in obese children. J Psychol 107:163, 172

Kincey J (1981) Internal-external control and weight loss in the obese. J Clin Psychol 37(1):100–103

Schachter S (1968) Obesity and eating. Science 161:751–756

CHAPTER 8

Common Elements in Dyscontrol Syndromes

Dyscontrol syndromes can be defined as the wide spectrum of behavioral disturbances (behavioral excesses) which are finally manifested as addictions. These syndromes are specifically food addiction which is manifested as obesity, thinness addiction which is manifested as anorexia nervosa (and bulimia), drug addiction (substance abuse), gambling, and activity addiction. These behavioral disturbances represent either the direct expression of the explosive, impulsive, disinhibited drive behavior, which is cyclic in nature, or the opposite – the inhibitory, controlled, rigidly sublimated behavior adhered to with compulsive rituality.

The threat of the impulse and the subsequent behavior can also exist only in fantasy, though countermeasures are still taken. Impulses can be pure drives, such as sex, the gratification of which is feared (threat of being a woman and the fear of fusion, of losing self-control, and of being abandoned). For women who experience difficulties in female identification, transformation is sometimes achieved by appearing as a rigidly, spiritually neutral being (anorexia nervosa).

The three main syndromes (obesity, drug addiction, and anorexia nervosa) tend towards somatic, physical solutions. The obese use direct drive satisfaction, drug addicts drive equivalents, and anorectics the inhibition and sublimation of drives. All dyscontrol syndromes are characterized by a striving for independence and autonomy – from both internal and external pressures. They also oscillate between various forms of concrete dependence and independence and include aspects of intrapsychic and interpersonal polarity (social aspects), also within their family life.

The essential elements in obesity, drug addiction, and anorexia nervosa are the same at the primary level (though they have different solutions). These include:

- morbid craving
- insatiability
- connections between oral intake and the feeling state
- deviant cues for interoceptive stimuli
- bodily expression of inner conflicts (affect discharged in uniform somatic response)

- behavioral excesses
- urgency of need satisfaction
- impulsivity, intolerance of tension or anxiety
- cyclic behavior (impulses) or repetition compulsion
- deviant libidinal expressions.

Deviant libidinal expressions include disturbances in sexual identity formation with either sublimation or drive equivalents and direct or indirect self-destructive behavior. There are also mythical or moralistic expressions, identifiable at various social and cultural levels, deverbalization and less symbolic creativity, and difficulty in mature object relations.

The difficulty in mature object relations can be expressed as dependence on (a) primary objects in the family, (b) transitional or delusional objects, (c) the own body as object, and (d) nonliving objects, i.e., food, which is personified, cathected, and thus treated as an object. Other characteristics include feelings of omnipotence achieved by mastery, denial and sublimation as main defences, dependence on the thrill of playing games with fate, and social conspicuousness.

In this chapter we will be looking at the various emotional, motivational, and psychosocial elements that play a role in these three major dyscontrol syndromes. A comparison of the three syndromes is given in Table 1.

Table 1. A comparison of the three major dyscontrol syndromes

Issues	Anorexia nervosa	Obesity	Drug dependence
Drives in general	Completely sublimated	Orality, regression of sex to orality	Drive equivalents
Hunger feeling	Ever present, but absolutely suppressed	Ever present	Stimulus hungry, suppressing it
Erotization (seductivity)	Resistance against any erotic meaning, even of food	Giving in to erotic meaning of food	Erotization of drug and procedure (skin, injection incorporation)
Mechanisms of incorporation	Fear and fantasies of incorporation	All-devouring	Incorporating body-alien elements
Supply	Danger of being full, false cues	Threat of being empty and depleted	Fill the missing, reduce control
Personification (object)	Food is object (personified)	Food is personified	Drug is personified
All have no real living objects and will animate nonliving objects			
Object relations	Almost complete avoidance, own body is hated object	Insulation layer symbolically keeps off contacts, fat body insulates from social contact (digust)	Drug turns into object equivalent just as drive turns into drive equivalent (quest for drugs)
Affect	Resomatized	Resomatized	Dedifferentiated

Table 1 (continued)

Issues	Anorexia nervosa	Obesity	Drug dependence
Tension-relaxation cycles	Tension most explicit	Elements of relaxation more felt	Vacillating cycles
Areas of attention	Fear of growth, tumescence, and inevitability	Fear of confrontation with body reality, the nude, and losing insulation	Fear of growing affect and emotion
Control	Model of overcontrol	Loss of control, letting go	Fight against control
Control by fantasies	Turning into neuter, stopping menstruation	Eating motivation: love and aggression	Chemical compounds work magic
Personality structure	Hysteric and borderline	Cyclothymic	Sociopathic or dissocial
Tolerance for suffering	Very high threshold	Large reserves for emergencies	Inability to tolerate suffering as such
Behavior mechanisms	Temper tantrums, self-destructive	In compulsive eaters some paroxysmal features ("14 and 6 per second spikes")	Often explosive behavior
Self-destructive	Directly	Indirectly	Both socially and self-destructive
Symbolize	The modest, sublimating Victorian	Enjoying, joyful, benevolent	Rebel, periphery of society
Mythical	The spiritual, sacred, victim	The flesh, hedonist	The criminal, the sinner
Social structure	Upper class	Middle class	Lower class, marginal
Historical	Victorian spinster	Plebeian, citizen	Modern, chemistry
Public image	Modest sublimating girl, against femininity and sex	The enjoying, "letting go" type	Fight against any control
Motivational	No wish to change	No strong motivation to change	Difficulty in changing
Social function	Victim arousing sympathy	Isolation, superficially sociable	Dissocial, digusting
Imitations	Caricature of medieval or Victorian purity	Caricature of obeying, feeding mother	Caricature of being a doctor (injecting)
Attitude to external (social stimuli)	Reduced body size, limited target for stimuli	Unreachable, more body insulation of the core	Stimuli less felt, perceived, apathetic due to drugs
Signals to environment	Don't touch, I am unnatural, not feminine, not human, half dead	Keep away, I am impulse-driven, animal-like, ugly	Keep away, I am explosive, a beast, a criminal
Time	Activity shortens time, fear of eternity	No ability to postpone or wait	Cannot wait or delay

Table 1 (continued)

Issues	Anorexia nervosa	Obesity	Drug dependence
Coping and defense	Displacement of affect, sublimation, denial, conversion, resomatization	Displacement, conversion	Neutralization, repression, suppression, manipulation
Motivation for treatment	None	Sometimes	When able to manipulate for gain
Painters' image	Modigliani	Rubens	Psychedelics
Doctors' attitude	Hard to understand, "crazy", endangering their lives	Not a real disease, matter of willpower	Fear and disgust, impotence

As can be seen from Table 1, the therapeutic ideology, strategy, and outcome have basic similarities in all three syndromes. Motivation for treatment does not originate usually with the patient; it normally stems from the surroundings – family, friends, or social or forensic institutions.

Therapy is difficult, as the ability for verbalization, symbolization, and introspection are all very low. Various kinds of social therapies are at present being applied. We physicians may be influenced by the patient's behavior and by our own feelings of incompetence, becoming reduced to using pharmacological treatment which in the end can make it even more difficult for the patient to verbalize, and can cause dependency. This is part of the general problem of the attitude of traditional medicine toward self-induced diseases, which we shall discuss in chapter 11 on Treatment.

CHAPTER 9

Psychodynamic Viewpoints of the Dyscontrol Syndromes and of Anorexia Nervosa in Particular

"Total abstinence is easier than perfect moderation."

St. Augustine: On the God of Marriage, c. 401 A.D.

The regressions we shall be treating here all happen in adolescence, a very sensitive period of human life, full of conflict. Adolescents are in a difficult transitional state, torn between a seductive upheaval of a libidinal id and a very severe superego. All this takes place in the internal world, while at the same time the adolescent is trying to deal with thought and action in the external world, to establish firm ego-functioning. Adolescents also experience weakness, vulnerability, and dependence as opposed to the image of the mighty parental figure.

The adolescent tries to deny his helplessness and his need for the omnipotent mother and father figures by acting in an exaggerated way in order to escape the pull back to regressive states. Very often this pull back is unavoidable, especially when something in the adolescent's former developmental stages was faulty.

We claim that the addictive syndromes, including anorexia nervosa, demonstrate an interplay between impulse and affect on the one hand, and various control mechanisms on the other, which, in the case of anorexia, has a compulsive element of overcontrol. In general, various states of regression can be discerned. There are several questions to be asked about such regressions: Why are affective responses controlled with such force? What is the social significance of this urgency and its almost unlimited mastering? What are the intrapsychic adaptive or maladaptive functions of such behavior? And why the somatization of feeling states?

Tomkins (1962) describes very early facial expressions as having "innate affect operating from birth." He divides them into positive and negative affects. We believe that structural physiological channelling of affects is there at birth, like grimaces, which are often interpreted as smiling responses, when the affective content will be there only much later. This appears to suggest that there are physiologic preparations for the later expression of affect. The earliest affective response of the baby is a global bodily response of incorporation or ejection. The triggering of affect expression is probably by way of information passing into the brain, a subcortical program, caused by stimuli and by its own triggering of affective expression.

In infancy "the dialectic communicative exchange between mother and child makes no distinction between affect response and perceptive-cognitive ordering" (Lichtenberg 1981). From birth on, the infant is delivered into the climate of the mother's affect. We know of early observable infantile reactions regarding awareness of approaching gratification (which is important in our context). This need for awareness and gratification will, in an abstract sense, grow into eagerness and fascination, which will be a common element in pleasant affects. At the same time, the frustration of such needs evokes the *Anlage* of anger. While mentioning gratification, we may already state that in these syndromes there is a certain playing with immediate gratification, and in some cases a conscious delay. It is a movement from the playful and the seductive to the challenge, the thrill, and the ecstasy. It is also the play between the immediate instinctual gratification and the later development of being able to delay such gratification to achieve a degree of sublimation compatible with reality, even to an exaggerated degree.

In obesity, for instance, there seems to be a giving in, an omission, of almost any control mechanisms. In drug abuse, there is deviant control and an acceptance of external incorporating matters. In anorexia, there is a very strict overcontrol mechanism, somewhat synchronous with the appearance of puberty.

When analyzing impulse-driven personalities, it appears that these people as children may have remained in an undifferentiated phase to an unusual degree, so that the ego proves inadequate to control the impulses and also unable to delay their direct gratification. As a consequence of this underdevelopment or fixation, other regressive elements may play a part.

We shall first discuss some points of ontogenetic development in order to study both developmental deficiencies and regressive states. Ontogenetic development constitutes a continuous spiral movement from direct explosive, discontinuous discharge of instinctual gratification toward a state of sublimation. Studies of social psychology specify very clear differences at both extremes. For example, Mischel (1966) based a series of studies on the choice preference for immediate smaller gratification versus delayed but more valuable rewards, two contrasting patterns of delay and impulsivity that have been conceptualized as extreme poles. At one extreme are those people who predominantly choose larger, delayed rewards or goals for which they must either wait or work. These individuals are more likely to be oriented toward the future and to plan carefully for distant goals. They are also likely to have high scores on ego-control measures, to have high achievement motivation, to be more trusting and socially responsible, to be brighter and more mature, to have a high level of aspiration, and to show less uncontrolled impulsivity. This extreme pattern resembles what has been called the Puritan character structure. Socioculturally, this pattern tends to be found more often in middle and upper socioeconomic classes and in highly achievement-oriented (Protestant ethic) cultures (Grim et al. 1968). This high level of competence is revealed by higher intelligence, more mature cognitive development, and a greater capacity for attention.

At the other extreme pole is the individual who predominantly prefers immediate gratification and rejects the alternative of waiting or working for larger delayed rewards or goals. Correlated with this is a greater concern with the immediate present than with the future, and greater impulsivity. Socioculturally, this pattern is found more often in the lower socioeconomic classes, in cultural groups in which achievement-orientation is low, and with indices of lesser social and cognitive competence. In these epure patterns, however, there may be compensatory devices and mechanisms of reversal and reaction formation which may cause similarities in explicit style and behavior, while being rooted in exactly opposite causes.

Anorectics are very much in a state of regression or are fixated in their development to an earlier stage, but in behavior they are very close to the pattern of pathologic tendency to delay immediate instinctual gratification. They usually belong to the higher socioeconomic classes and are of superior intelligence, and can therefore easily imitate those in their class in their normative behavior. They have, on a superficial level, persons with whom they can identify and circles to adapt to. But basically, and primarily, they are impulse-ridden, insatiably hungry, explosive characters threatened by their own anxiety. Therefore, they "choose" to overcontrol their basic needs in a specific way that they have learned and have partly adapted to this overcontrol. This adaptation may be in the form of counterphobic mechanisms or other compensations which are used to get over their deep-seated fears of invasion into body.

Returning to the study of the various developmental axes, growth can be seen as a movement from a state of symbiosis with the mother toward a state of individuation. Another axis would be the emotional need for a feeling of closeness to the world of objects as one pole, and the desire to be remote from such a world, to keep a distance from the living object world, on the other pole. With this developmental trend, however, there are varying stages of movement in healthy subjects between the two poles and they do not show signs of arrest at any stage. Even in some states of part-symbiosis with other objects, a state of dual unity may be achieved in the healthy adult in the service of the ego. States such as love, mystical experiences, the situation of the dedicated master and devoted pupil, as well as that between hypnotist and the hypnotized subject are known and have been thoroughly analyzed. Therefore, antinomy can be seen between closeness versus detachment, and symbiosis versus individuation.

This makes it clear that every individual has the potential ability to "construct" a wide variety of behavior patterns which can be used for self-control depending on the personality style, its adaptability, and the quality and intensity of the imagined threat. Such bipolarity does not necessarily have deviant significance. Duality in life is essential.

In intrapersonal issues reality and fantasy are not opposed, but are in fact two poles of the same axis. As a result, spontaneity (or even impulsivity) and sublimated behavior can be in constant movement and therefore not in any rigidly frozen position. Even symmetry and asymmetry may be opposed qualities which together can creat positive tensions. Furthermore, development moves from random responses, the involvement of basic vegetative processes and primary process thinking toward coordinated motor action, to desomatization and secondary process thinking.

Development will be in the direction of desomatization, and verbalization of affect. The possibility of verbal emotional expression, symbol formation, and the utilization of words in cognition have to do with maturational factors and therefore also depend on former anatomical channelling and physiologic changes. In regressive states, however, there will be a return to earlier mechanisms in some of these factors achieved by development. Regressive states of mind are determined by a multiplicity of factors. They can be evoked by severe stress, exhaustion, illness, or intoxication, and seen in drug-induced states, extreme passion and finally also in creative art, and as such will be used, as mentioned, in the service of the ego.

Psychoanalytic literature on regression used to relate to drive activity and discharge, to the functioning of the ego and to superego aspects. Expressions of regression are attempts at resomatization, deverbalization, and dedifferentiation between the concrete and the symbolic. There is not only a dedifferentiation of affect, but even a regression to bodily-bound sensations. If there are affects they seem closely connected with bodily feelings. (Progressive development from bodily sensations into emotions have to do with cognitive development and its complexity, with the ability to abstract, aided by the autonomous nervous system.) Thus, in the case of severe regression, sensations are more prevalent than complex emotions.

In order to understand developmental failures or regressions, let us look at the differentiation of self and object representation, and the related ego defenses, as well as adaptive mechanisms in general. Intrapsychic structures develop through the slow progressive differentiation of the self representation from the object representation and with it the development of a certain style of defense mechanism. A developmental failure along this continuum results in an arrest in the differentiation of both the self and the object representation, and in their related ego functions as well as in the process of desomatization. If the arrest occurs in the symbiotic phase, the self and object representations are fused and the person's ego defenses are splitting and projecting. This results in poor ego boundaries and poor reality testing, as well as delusional thinking.

There seems to be an early phase in life during which failure can particularly occurs. However, as development is a continuum, the arrest can occur at practically any point. This is also true of symbiosis and the separation-individuation phase. These might include fantasies of the good or bad mother, but even more the wish to reunite with, not to lose the mother, the wish to fuse with her or her substitute, often the father. This can be seen as an awareness of approaching gratification, as an eagerness or fascination of this wished-for fusion, and as an object addiction.

In cases in which the arrest occurs somewhat earlier on the continuum there may be a symbol formation of an earlier and part-mother substitute, namely the transitional object. In the specific case of anorexia this transitional object, animated and personified, is food itself. Diverse incoming sensations and afferent or emotional signals are being channelled into a single, unidirectional response, namely, to the gastrointestinal tract alone. This seems to be an underdevelopment of the abiltiy to react to differential stimuli with differential responses. However, it may also be a limitation at the level of experience.

In these personalities there is a split in the ego and denial due to overwhelming flooding affects. Consequently, an attempt is made to reestablish mastery by magical thinking and action (i.e., drugs). Relief is gained by pleasure and by a sense of power, but then remorse and shame take over. There is also a split in the superego, and as a result these personalities indulge in uncontrolled instinctual gratification with the implicit, though unconscious, objective of defeating the parental introjection which has been incorporated into the ego and superego, more as an alien body than as an integrated part of the personality.

As we have stated, when food is the object representation, the imagined substitute of the mother – and possibly her negation – it can be devoured and thus incorporated. In this interaction both oral and anal elements play a part. Filling and emptying, fulfilling and ejecting – the subject-object relationship is turned into an autistic game. The "yes" and "no" are seductive elements, and they turn into almost obsessional cyclic mechanisms in the service of gaining total control of the object. Control here is a useful mechanism against strong, overwhelming, threatening drives, or the feeling of inner chaos which may be caused by such a threat. In that sense, strong control is a countermeasure, and as such may of course also exceed "intended" proportions. Eroticism in general, sex in particular, and the fact of being a woman are very severe threats to existence in anorectics, who avoid all connection with these issues. Therefore, the anorectic tries to turn into a neutral, sexually unpretentious being, not only by avoiding a female appearance, but also by being able to suppress omnipotently any drive, even the most vital one, hunger. By controlling hunger the anorectic is able to prove her ability to suppress less vital drives, such as sex. This omnipotent feeling makes the anorectic believe she is the only woman who can stop her menstruation at will. The anorectic also plays the role of the one who cannot be controlled. She acts out infantile fantasies of omnipotence, of being master of life and death (or of being possessed by the devil). She is the ascetic who can control her body as an object and her needs may turn into a game of being possessed, of being a witch. By taking on the imagery of a witch the anorectic may demonstrate the paradox of the unwanted sexual woman who can control not only herself, but can also even change the size of her body parts. She is possessed by an idea, and the putting of that idea into reality. She can sustain life in spite of being on the verge of dying.

The other "game" practiced by anorectics involves a kind of severe, almost ascetic, Spartan behavior, which comes close to the classic religious forms of masochistic and ascetic behavior. It is a means of taming the "soft," feminine body. Through asceticism a reduction in pain sensitivity is developed, as well as a relative insensitivity to cold and hunger sensations. It is seen as a way to better adaption or resistance to environmental nonliving influences, resulting in the ability to live a tougher life. Altogether, this produces a heightening of transcendent dimensions and a reduction of physical sensitivity and awareness. The rigid belief in a split between body and mind motivates some anorectics to attempt to crush the strong, demanding body in order to enhance the weak spirit (i.e., the spirit works better when fasting).

In order to minimize the influence of somatic elements, sensory input is reduced and made less important in the process of perception – awareness – conception. For instance, reduction of sensory hunger stimulus through fasting enhances intellectual, central mechanisms, since pain stimuli are minimized or denied somewhere in this chain of perception. Also, as mentioned, environmental temperature stimuli are less disturbing. Therefore, denial can be seen as a psychological defense or adaptive mechanism which is strong and vital enough to influence the whole life of the organism. But one also has to consider to what extent denial is an expression of real slowing or dampening of physiological processes.

Another game used is mockery of society and the law: drugs used instead of food by drug abusers, or no food instead of food by anorectics. Anorectics do not refuse food altogether, as psychotics do, and are not suspicious or paranoid, but they rigidly insist on low intake. Their thin bodies are the guarantees that they are winning the fight against passive surrender to food.

Anorectics also display a return to the neutral instead of the differentiated gender – "I am still a fetus," i.e., not able to leave the uterus of the family. It is as if they have not experienced individuation and/or differentiation.

Puberty brings about new experiences of a changing body. It is not only growth, but differentiation. With the physical changes, a sense of being different and often alienated from the former concept of oneself is experienced. The more neutral body build of the preadolescent is sometimes retained by a deviation of the body image. This bodily change seems unacceptable to the anorectic. Growth generates the wish, at least partly, to be grown up and belong to adult society. Growth also causes fascination and excitement. In primitive people, as in the child, it is believed that food contributes to change. Ingestion and incorporation are probably the most early mechanisms known to change body shape.

Universal themes in human life have a greater impact if they are ambiguous. Myths and fairy tales thrive on such subjects. Change of size of the human body, of its shape, or at least parts of its body (often a *pars pro toto* symbol) is a common theme with variations in fairy tales and in folklore. From small to big, from big to exploding, or changing back, making the irreversible reversible. Often, these changes happen in ecstatic states, in dreams, when sleeping, or in wishing states. Fascination and excitement about growth are universal, as also is excitement over differences in size and changes as such, for instance, pregnancy, breast growth, tumescence, and swelling of various organs. Growth is not under our willpower and control.

Human growth and development, the creation of human life, the growth of organs, filling space and fulfilling, as well as ejection and evacuation arouse curiosity, fear, and ambiguity. In the same way that it may be exciting for the young healthy female to get pregnant, to watch and enjoy the bodily changes taking place, it may also be exciting for the adolescent girl to watch her first bodily sexual change but this with anxiety and concern for the expected and the feared. It may also be exciting for the not-so-healthy female, disturbed emotionally and in body-image perception, to produce a self-induced, creative change to a nonmenstruating, nonpregnant, "nonwoman," – a viable skeleton. This can be seen as a mastery-effort to overcome change, by actively trying to control the differentiation of growth into a woman. It is the inevitability of change from the undifferentiated child into the differentiated woman that these girls are so afraid of, and which they therefore actively try to master by regulating and changing their life-style in such an extreme way.

In the anorectic this behavior can cause fascination with her own omnipotence and with the ways she has developed for dealing with what she feels are anxiety-provoking changes. Therefore, in order to be in control, she overcontrols this growth behavior, tries to reverse these "natural phenomena," and finally enjoys her mastery. The anorectic desires to return to a neuter state and thus wishes to be more ethereal and spiritual; at the same time she can continue to live concretely in this world, albeit at the limits of viability. From time to time (in bulimic stages), there may be a pleasant experience, or even an ecstasy of lust, in the giving in to impulses to swallow everything. Excitement will develop from the pleasure of pain, of withholding, of ascetiscism, of the God-like controlling of all that is earthly and secular.

In the typically obsese, there might be the excitement of changes felt to be self-induced without, however, having to fight impulses or drives. These individuals can passively watch the change in size and volume and enjoy it. There is, of course, also the element of not being approached and bothered, the need to isolate the core personality, and the insulating layer of fat which seems to be both a need and defense. In contrast, the drug abuser, by the intake of the drug, may experience a change in physical appearance and body shape. This keeps the drug abuser apart from social reality, apathy being the dominant emotional state. The liberation of the body and its autonomy is concretized by insensitivity to pain, to cold, to hunger, and to sexual needs. But real hunger for love is betrayed by the importance that people with dyscontrol syndromes attach to food, and sometimes to sex, in their drawings, dreams, and fantasies.

In our clinical experience we observed an interesting phenomenon in four anorectic girls, aged between 17–23 years. All of them had the habit of eating an apple when lying in bed in the evening, claiming it helped them to fall asleep. It was the only time and opportunity to be without tension and in a state of tranquillity. They enjoyed holding the round apple and biting into it and chewing. Could the apple possibly symbolize the round feminine form in contrast to their own "squareness," or was it the mother being devoured, or at least the breast being eaten up and incorporated? The apple may be connected with the biblical garden of Eden as a symbol which derives from paradisic pleasures, or in an ambiguous way it may symbolize the plight of curiosity, knowledge, and finally sublimation. According to Genesis, after eating the fruit from the tree of knowledge humans began to be aware of good and evil, of drive needs and conscience. Sublimation was thus initiated.

Food in general has an obvious concrete element, as well as the symbolic, the developmental (concrete-abstract), and the mythical elements that are close to the symbolic. Let us summarize some examples of language referring to the use of food and growth:

- The mother tells the child, "The more you eat, the bigger you will grow, the stronger you will be," or "If you don't eat, you will grow thinner and thinner, until nothing will be left of you." (Such "educational" threats are often found in children's books.)
- "I can exist without food, like I can without love."
- "I do not have to swallow in order to feel."
- "If I eat, I shall swell up without end, and finally explode" (have no control).
- In love: "I shall eat you up."
- In obesity: "I always have to have something in my mouth," or "I eat, although I am not hungry, but later I might be" (eating as hoarding), or "Today I deserved my food" (it was a bad day), or "Eating is insured pleasure, I do not have any other pleasures in life."

Appetite on the one hand, and eroticism on the other (in contrast to hunger and sex) are the more refined elements and need the ability to discriminate – to select and sublimate. Sexual abstinence is like solitary confinement. The body becomes the substitute for external objects and therefore undergoes a resomatization process. The external world is decathected, and the body becomes the arena of all happenings. It is like returning to a primary state of somatopsychic entity.

Affective responses and reactions occur within the gastrointestinal system which is made to swallow or not swallow the object. Pleasure or abstinence from pleasure are also pressured into the system, unlike any other autonomic, physiological function in the body. The movements of the gastrointestinal tract can be speeded up, slowed down, braked, and reversed, and its contents can be changed, minimized, or exaggerated. Control over this autonomous system is so developed that the system seems to adapt to this strict control. The extreme use and abuse of this system, such as induced retromovement, the great abuse of laxatives, or the lowering of secretory activity seem to undergo adaptive processes, so that there is no physiological rebellion, as might happen to other organ systems when abused. If there are rebellious (pathological) reactions they are relatively subtle. So we are able to postulate that the anorectic is successful in being in almost absolute control of her own autonomous organ system. It is a victory over instinctual demands. It may be worthwhile to note here that anorexia and bulimia lie on the same axis but at different poles.

Food, in contrast to the body, is animated and changed into a living object. Being an object, it works like a drug and is seen to be both seductive and seducible. It is refused, fought for, or accepted. It is belittled in its value but magnified and exaggerated in its concrete form and shape. Anorectics measure, obsessively control, and finally eat food – lovingly, impulsively, tenderly or aggressively. By not eating, the anorectic denies her impulse to destroy the incorporated primary object (repressing cannibalistic impulses). The remaining symptoms are thus constant hunger and a constant struggle against it.

This is almost a caricature, in an autistic way, of social interaction. But it also serves manipulative issues in the family. Elements of swallowing and incorporating can include behavior of a more applied type. Namely, on a higher level of "incorporation," it would mean a refusal to learn or read. Or, in line with bulimic behavior, it would mean a greedy absorption of books and other visual (edible) objects such as paintings – again an incorporation or swallowing.

As a matter of fact, the behavior we mentioned is concerned only with nonliving objects, which can be handled without threat or danger. Also nonautonomous, even central functions not only remain but are definitely reinforced. So, sublimation is enacted – the striving toward the intellectual and the purely spiritual, toward the transcendent and the sublime.

In drug abuse, similar mechanisms are at work. Both drug abuse and anorexia show a great body cathexis as well as fear of overwhelming body needs and functions. The main difference is that drug abusers use drugs in place of food, sex is decathected, and substances from the outside devoured. Drugs are substituted for objects, and strict control mechanisms are used to manage otherwise autonomous functions such as satiety, hunger, pain, and temperature.

Time Aspects

Anorectics exhibit intricate and implicit disturbances of time perception. Their experience of growing up within a span of time is certainly incomplete. They behave either like infants who have not grown up, or as elderly people whose interest is focused only on their bodies. At the same time anorectics act as if their bodies do not exist. Theirs is a fear of the irreversibility of time or of the irrevocable nature of growing up. Anorectics want to stop the passage of time; they want to remain children, guarded from life within the safe, denying family group.

There is often a fear of time advancing, as if time were an internal monster. This fear can increase when growth is uncontrolled, as with the development of sexual characteristics in puberty. It is a fear that with the progression of time the body, when being fed, will grow continuously. The limitlessness of time, like the eternity of Nirvana or of paradise, so characteristic of the id, is very threatening. Repetitive behavior may be an unconscious device to return to perinatal cyclical behavior and thereby to break the limitlessness of time. To this time aspect also belongs the fear of the inevitable monthly period. Simone de Beauvoir described the traumatic shock of the menarche in her book *The Memories of a Dutiful Daughter.* Though not every girl experiences the onset of menstruation as a shock, those who are obsessed with every indication of their femininity may feel the need to do away with it. The inevitability of its monthly, periodic occurrance is seen as a losing battle against an invincible body. This loss of power, which is symbolized by loss of blood, is a constant reminder of being a woman; these losses can be arrested either by pregnancy or by ceasing to be a woman, by changing the body. This need to cease being a woman is reinforced by the role feminine sexuality plays in our culture. As Baker-Miller (1978) states: "The woman's territory is essentially that of man's unresolved problems. Issues with which the dominant culture has never come to terms, e.g., sexuality, death, emotions – these are handed over to the domain of women. Thus, man is enabled to exorcise a demon of his own by punishing woman for her sexuality."

Chodorow (1974) suggests an interesting theory of feminine identity-formation and general developmental steps, as compared with the male. She believes that issues of dependency and relationships on the whole are experienced differently by women and men. Chodorow claims that, for boys, separation and individuation are critically tied to gender identity since separation from the mother is essential for the development of masculinity. For girls, issues of femininity or feminine identity do not depend on the achievement of separation from the mother or on the progress of individuation. "Since masculinity," she states, "is defined through separation, while femininity is defined through attachment, male gender identity is threatened by intimacy while female gender identity is threatened by separation. Thus, males tend to have difficulty with relationships, while females tend to have problems with identification." Thus, in regard to the body there may be a neutralization and depersonalization which can result in a kind of dissociative mechanism in which the awareness of hunger and satiety are separated from this depersonalized body.

Hunger

Hunger in infancy sets the model for later addictive behavior. It has a quality of urgency and irresistibility, which tolerates no delay and no disappointment. Withdrawal from any morbid craving has its model in the weaning process of infancy. Whatever is taken in (by whatever mode of incorporation) is a form of feeding in response to some form of hunger. Hunger, however, can also be a need for warmth, closeness, and body contact. A denial of this general hunger can be seen as a process of hibernation, of temporarily retreating from the world. This denial of general hunger, this bodily winter sleep, is a rejection of the need for human closeness, for support, and for differentiation. The impact of external sources on the body is reduced, with the resulting ability to tolerate pain and extreme temperatures more easily. The senses of smell and taste are reduced. But, in contrast to real hibernation, reserves are not filled and energy is not stored. Energy is delibidinized, neutralized and used in a completely intellectual, spiritual context only[1].

The anorectic's extreme need for control is connected with the period of adolescence, a time of extreme polarities, of the need for purity, sublimation, and liberation of the body as a rebellion against drive strength. The anorectic continues to express this rebellion. With advancing years, however, this extreme control is needed less because of a natural decline in drive strengths.

The strange, almost paradoxical behavior of anorectics – namely, feeling full, active, and well after having eaten little – may have other sources. It may be the result of faulty learning from childhood, or actually the development of false or inverted cues. For anorectics, a void signifies control, satisfaction, and activity. With eating, there is fullness, distention, a fear of lack of boundaries, of not being able to stop, and a deep sense of guilt. Emptiness therefore causes pleasure.

In general, the female has a need to fill a sensed inner space. On a higher, more abstract level this may mean fulfillment. The normal woman has an awareness of her inner space. In contrast, this sense of inner space among anorectics is repressed and seemingly nonexistent. Therefore, there can be no pleasure in filling such an empty space if it cannot be sensed.

The need for extreme self-control is the major characteristic of anorectics. It is probably the only possible reaction to their complex state. This reaction can lead to a certain dynamic equilibrium. Although the state itself may be seen as pathologic, like so many other disturbed reactions it is able to keep the organism

---

[1] Anorexia does occur in some animal species and is predictable. The eating patterns are not the result of changes in food availability. Hibernating animals begin hibernating even when food is available. The regulation of body weight has then been set under different rules depending on the seasonal cycle. The red jungle fowl (female) sits on the egg, and during the 20 days of incubation food intake is reduced to 20% of baseline levels and body weight falls by 20% (Sherry 1981).

in a state of functionality, albeit a reduced one. This reaction goes on continuously as an interplay of inhibition and disinhibition, impulsivity and compulsive control, symbiotic behavior and individuation, and other polarities. This interplay seems to be in the service of the survival of the individuum. It does not seem to really matter if that "milieu" was caused primarily by internal, external or mixed elements. Though it can be created by purely affective states and their regressive dimensions, and by endocrine correlates (or reinforced by the administration of drugs), the interplay with the self-control reaction remains the same.

All dyscontrol syndromes exhibit not only the control and various mastering mechanisms of the present, but with it the need for the thrill of controlling the future, life and death. In anorexia this seems like a manipulative game, a bond with the devil, a Faustian element. This Faustian element, as viewed by Stent (1978), is man locked in endless strife with his world to overcome obstacles, controlling and actually not being in control, the resulting conflict in his mind being the very essence of existence. By reaching for the infinite he is never satisfied.

The regressive elements, together with rigid control, are expressed by the anorectic through resomatization, deverbalization, and dedifferentiation of the concrete and the symbolic. More archaic devices such as splitting, dissociation, depersonalization, and animation or personalization of food are also used. Basically, there seems to be a failure of separation and individuation, which can be observed in the fusion with parents and the family, and in the anxiety concerning growing up and leaving home. This failure of separation and individuation can sometimes be expressed by a certain synchronicity of mood swings with one of the parents.

Other defects seems to be inherent in a disturbed development of emotions. The usual development of emotions from bodily sensations and their admixture with a complexity of cognitive elements, associations, memories, thoughts, etc., seems to be interrupted and disrupted in anorectics. As with other regressive elements, sensation seems to be more prevalent than complex emotions. Some emotions, such as anger, tension, anxiety, and even happiness or euphoria are definitely connected with and expressed by physical sensations. In these cases, different incoming sensational or emotional signals are channelled into a single, unidirectional response, exclusively to the gastrointestinal tract.

In contrast, for the obese, the obvious wish could be the thrill and pleasure of giving in and manipulating the avoidance of responsibility. In drug abuse, the thrill of seduction and resistance against it plays a large role, as well as the need to rebel against society. All three syndromes show certain biological correlates in adjacent brain areas, especially those concerned with functions of hunger, appetite, satiety, sexual behavior, satisfaction, temperature control, and pain sensitivity. These areas are also represented by functional systems of neuroamines and are interconnected with neuropeptides. It is therefore possible to speculate on the significance of the biological mechanisms of inhibition and disinhibition, of charge and discharge, of control and superposition, and whether they are, in some way, mirror images or correlates of similar psychological mechanisms.

The influence of the father as a major contributing factor in anorexia nervosa has not been fully investigated. The studies which do exist usually rely on patient material without control cases, and present little that is substantiated or original. Nevertheless, these studies often show the interesting phenomenon of anorectics experiencing mood swings which are synchronous with those of the father. It can therefore be assumed that the Oedipal relationship and fantasy relating to the father is more important than has been assumed. In our studies we have seen three cases involving almost open incestuous father-daughter relationships. It seems to be the image of the seductive father which can initiate anorectic behavior, with the patient desiring to devour and thereby incorporate him. In turn, the daughter must punish herself for this sexual desire, and this punishment is carried out by self-inflicted starvation, which makes the patient unfeminine. This also punishes the father, by showing him what kind of female he is attracted to. In addition, we have frequently heard anorectic patients mention that their fathers have a similar, usually moody personality. Other authors (Becker 1980; Reid 1986) have stressed the importance of the father as a factor in determining anorectic behavior.

In addition to our own experience concerning incest fantasies and the role of the anorectic's father, Caroll et al. (1980) suggests that incest, or rather the fantasy of incest, results in the development of a punitive conscience in the victim, which under stress overwhelms the weak ego defenses and triggers self-injury. Profiles of anorectic and incest groups are similar, and both are different from control groups. The fact that anorectics are frequently oblivious to both their psychological and physical damage is clearly reflected in the ego defense mechanisms of denial and repression (Scott and Thoner 1986).

Finally, as a resume of assumed dynamics in the development of this syndrome, we believe that the following issues are to be considered coping mechanisms in their widest sense:

1. Reduction of sensory input at various levels; with it, reduction of excitability and with that, increase in motor output
2. Resistance to external and internal stimuli, overcompensation, negating, denying, and even reversal of affect
3. Sublimation as a conspicuous issue as well as obsessive-compulsive repetitive behavior
4. Personalization (animation) of non-living matter
5. Dedifferentiation of affect
6. Deverbalization
7. Resomatization with special stress on the gastrointestinal system
8. Object relations remaining in an autistic state; omnipotence feelings may prevail, and as a result it seems to be a fake relationship with a fake object.

The following polarities exist on various axes in anorectics:

bodily	spiritual
full	empty
fat	thin
concrete	ethereal, abstract
wish	refusal of, anxiety
drive	control
impulsive	compulsive
desomatization (maturity)	resomatization (regression)
verbalization	deverbalization
feminine	defeminization (neutral)
impulsive drive behavior	sublimation
factual irreversibility	imagined reversibility

Family Dynamics

In absolute numbers more studies have been carried out on intrapsychic dynamics than on intrafamilial dynamics. It is therefore not easy, and from a statistical point of view hardly reliable, to generalize from the studies made. Nevertheless, there are certain conceptual conclusions that can be made from the studies of therapists and researchers who have been working with families in many different areas.

The family approach concentrates on understanding the dynamics of the family system, their communications, and alliances. One of the most important early researchers in this field was Haley (1963), who claimed in his theoretical formulations that aspects of communication have to be understood in order to comprehend the role of a patient in the family context. He pointed out that it is impossible not to communicate and not to respond to a communication, and that every communication involves at least two levels (content and relationship definition). Selvini-Palazzoli (1963) also saw the family as a system and not just as a sum of its parts. She claimed that within a self-regulatory process the family is a rule-governed system. This system has a "rule of rules" in that it is forbidden to make comments or to metacommunicate about the rules. She also showed clearly that a family is a system of transformation. In a psychotherapeutic study her research on 12 families with anorectic members led her to reach the conclusion that family members freely display drama and suffering. Family members qualify their communications coherently, both verbally and nonverbally. However, rejection of messages by other members is frequent. There seems to be a problem of leadership; when there is a reluctance to assume leadership on the part of one of the parents and a wrong decision is made, blame is shifted onto another family member.

Selvini-Palazzoli (1963) also looked at the problem of alliances within the family unit, which of course exists in every family. She noted that family members seem to see any alliance between two members as a betrayal of a third. Finally, she claims that behind a facade of respectability and unity in the partnership, there is a great deal of disillusionment between marriage partners which is covered up by massive denial. It is also quite well-substantiated that each parent feels compassion for the anorectic daughter, but then expresses disillusionment when this is frustrated. Selvini-Palazzoli concludes that in families with an anorectic member, there is such a general rejection of communication that the rejection of food seems to be in keeping with the accepted style of interaction within the family. Similar impressions have been expressed by Minuchin (1970) and Barcai (1971).

We ourselves found that within these families there is a great deal of conflict avoidance and denial. It is as if the anorectic member, by concentrating all attention on her own problems, keeps the parents from expressing their own difficulties. She is the enfant terrible, the cause of constant anxiety and concern, a continuous threat, and a source of guilt for the family.

In contrast to present-day permissiveness, particularly of upper middle class families, anorectics present an archaic symbol of Victorian values – of inhibitions, modesty, and of course of sublimatory strength. Anorectic girls provoke implicitly hidden anger in the parents, since they do not socialize as others do, they insist on remaining in a state of dependency in the framework of the family, and do not want to leave it in order to grow up. On the other hand, the anorectic is also rebelling against accepted norms within the family structure (especially at family meetings which usually take place at meals), thereby showing the other side of their ambiguity, namely, stressing their autonomy in a negative sense. In the Oedipal situation, since the anorectic cannot compete as a woman with the mother for the father, she denies her feminine identity while at the same time impressing on the father her other nonfeminine attributes. And, as we stated above, there might be an incestuous bond, initiated explicitly by the father, and carried on by the anorectic, who then punishes him by "drying out" as a woman, thereby showing him the horrifying skeleton she really is.

The incidence of anorexia with respect to geographic areas, socioeconomic levels, and professional groups is interesting and may express and strengthen some of the assumptions on etiology, or at least some common dynamic elements. For example, it has been stressed again and again that anorexia is basically a Western, upper middle class phenomenon which usually affects highly intelligent and active women. Indeed, it would be difficult to imagine that this syndrome, which contains elements of rebellion, could exist among the poor and hungry in India. Nevertheless, in recent years, anorexia seems to be less a Western upper middle class phenomenon; we have seen three anorectics from Middle Eastern Jewish cultures whose intelligence, as measured by psychological tests, was not particularly high. Anorectic behavior does seem to be more prevalent in certain professions, especially among ballet dancers or professional female athletes. These women exhibit a morbid fear of fatness. Nevertheless, it is hard to imagine that they do not feel feminine.

I must mention here the interesting personal observations submitted to me by an ethnologist who worked for many years in Nepal researching the initiation rites, shaman activity, and other cultural activities of the inhabitants. Interestingly enough, he observed that many of the women scientists carrying out research in that area became anorectic and that many returned to their own countries for that reason. This phenomenon was part of a general experience of emotional problems and symptoms experienced by both the men and women scientists, due to the difficult conditions under which they worked. They had no knowledge of the languages of the area and were considered dumb by the natives. Everyone worked alone and lived in almost absolute isolation. Nevertheless there still was no privacy to speak of.

It was assumed that those who went to work in Nepal had some sort of rebellious attitude toward their own society, were somewhat adventurous in character, and were highly ambitious. In Nepal, everyone felt tense and libido was very low in both men and women. Many women, especially those in the age group 20–30 years became very thin, resembling real anorectics. Some of them had to return to their own countries because of these difficulties, which they attributed to severe stress.

Offhand, it seems that this reaction by the women scientists was a defensive maneuver to control the pleasurable experience of eating since no other pleasurable behavior was possible. That this anorectic behavior and anything to do with feminine identification is at least doubtful. It seems as if it was a specific reaction to an unbearable stress situation in which these women felt trapped, isolated, and vulnerable. It is as if by overcontrolling intake they could defend themselves from further harm. Other external factors, for example atmospheric and climatic conditions, may have had an influence. Social and sensory isolation also may have caused depressive reactions, which resulted in loss of weight.

Summarizing the assessment of the developing dynamics in these states, it seems appropriate to make an estimate of ego functions, their strength, and their weaknesses. We are quite aware of the fact that there may be major differences and variations concerning the severity of the syndrome and that adaptive compensatory mechanisms, secondarily following certain deficiencies in ego functions, will be mobilized.

However, we would still like to categorize those various ego functions, and understand which are weakened, or disturbed in anorectics. We take up L. Bellak's scheme, which has proved useful in understanding indications of psychotherapy and its success through out a number of years (Bellak and Sheehy 1976). He distinguishes 12 major ego functions, which will be described here and differentially analyzed with regard to anorexia nervosa.

We must be aware of the fact that there might be uneven ego development, so that certain functions mature earlier than others. In addition, only certain ego functions may be affected and "damaged" by a certain regressive element while others may compensate.

Immature Ego Functions

Let us examine ego functions, one by one (Bellak and Hurvich 1969) including a new one, time concept.

1. Reality Testing. The ability to differentiate between inner and outer stimuli – a continuous selective scanning and matching of contemporary percepts against past percepts and ideas – is called reality testing.

In anorexia nervosa space is identical inside and outside, with no clear borders, and internal growth may be limitless. Body image is connected with a false space concept and connected with a split-off concept of the body, an object by itself.

The body seems to be a golem under control, devoid of need (drive) manifestations: no skin sensitivity, no fat, no monthly period, no breasts, no pain, no appetite, and no hunger. The body is just a gastrointestinal tract, the most primitive mouth-anus connection. Its only isolated function involves being fed, incorporation, rejection and ejection. The body is depersonalized.

2. Time Concept. With no experience of growing up, there is no realistic time concept. There is also a fear of irreversibility. The drive is endless, (not cyclic as in animals), and the drive power is therefore limitless in time and extent; like an internal monster, it can grow and grow immensely when uncontrolled.

3. Judgment. In anorectics comprehension and appraisal of hypothetical and real situations, and contemplated future are quite good.

4. Sense of Reality of the World and of Self. Self-boundaries, derealization, and self-esteem are disturbed in anorectics. Self-esteem is very much decreased.

5. Regulation and Control of Drives, Affects, Impulses. In the controlling of mechanisms in an adaptive way, the anorectic exhibits overcontrol of drives and of impulses.

6. Object Relations. In reactions to persons in the present, concerning closeness and distance, the anorectic has very distant, disturbed object relations.

7. Thought Processes. The anorectic has a well-preserved adaptiveness in memory concentration and attention, and has the ability to conceptualize, with language reflecting a primary or secondary process.

8. Adaptive Regression in the Service of the Ego. The ability of the ego to initiate a partial, temporary, and controlled lowering of its own functions in the furtherance of its interests (promoting adaptation) is known as adaptive regression. This is disturbed in the anorectic and causes a high level of fear.

9. Defensive Functioning. By controlling the emergence of anxiety-arousing or other dysphoric psychic factors (such as ego-alien instinctual wishes, affects, thought, and perception which conflict with the demands of the superego and reality), defensive functioning contributes to adaptation. Any function may at specific times be erected defensively against any other ego function.

In anorectics, this defensive functioning is very well preserved. One of their major defenses is denial of developmental demands by holding on to infantile family interactions through their eating patterns.

10. Stimulus Barrier. Thresholds and responses to stimuli both contribute to adaptation by the organism's potential for responding to high, average or low sensory input so that optimal homeostasis is maintained. This determines how resilient a person is, or how he readapts after stress. Only inanimate stimuli are involved, with various sensory modalities. In anorectics, this adaptation is very much disturbed.

11. Autonomous Functioning. Perception, memory, and language (involving intentionality, concentration, attention, hearing, vision, speech, productivity, motor development, and expression) are aspects of autonomous functioning that can be affected by the intrusion of conflict, ideation, affect and/or impulse. This functioning is disturbed in anorectis.

12. Synthetic-Integrative Functioning. The ability to integrate contradictory values, affect, behavior, and role conflicts with flexible consistency is disturbed in anorectics.

13. Mastery–Competence. In anorectics, the mastery-competence element is seemingly well-handled, but in actual fact the overdoing and overvaluation of this element shows disturbance.

An estimation of the various ego functions gives us some idea of ego resilience or vulnerability and of the strength and forces together with therapeutic motivations and efforts.

References

Baker-Miller J (1978) Toward a new psychology of women. Penguin, London

Barcai A (1971) Family therapy in the treatment of anorexia nervosa. Am J Psychiatry 3:286–290

Becker H (1980) Die Vater-Tochter-Beziehung in der Familiendynamik bei anorexia-nervosa Patientinnen. Nervenarzt 51:568–572

Bellak L, Hurvich M (1969) A systematic study of ego-functions. J Nerv Ment Dis 148(6):571–573

Bellak L, Sheehy M (1976) Broad role of ego function assessment. Am J Psychiatry 133 (11): 1259–1264

Caroll J, Shaffer C, Spensley J, Abramowitz SL (1980) Family experience of self-mutilating patients. Am J Psychiatry 137:852–853

Chodorow N (1974) Family structure and feminine personality. In: Rosaldo MZ, Lamphere L (eds) Women, culture and society. Stanford University Press, Stanford

Grim DF, Kohlberg L, White SH (1968) Some relationship between conscience and attentional processes. J Pers Soc Psychol 8:239–252

Haley J (1963) Strategies of psychotherapy. Grune and Stratton, New York

Klineberg SL (1968) Future time perspective and the preference for delayed reward. J Pers Soc Psychol 8:253–257

Lichtenberg J (1981) The empathic mode of perception and alternative vantage points for psychoanalytic work. Psychoanal Inquiry 1(3):329–356

Minuchin S (1970) The use of an ecological framework in the treatment of a child. In: Anthoni J, Koupernik C (eds) The child in his family. Wiley, New York

Mischel W (1966) Theory and research on the antecedents of self-imposed delay of reward. In: Maher BA (ed) Progress in experimental personality research 3. Academic, New York, pp 85–132

Reid JC (1986) Der lebenswichtige Vater. Symptome der anorexia nervosa bei unterschiedlichen psychischen Krankheiten als Ausdruck der Vaterproblematik. Anal Psychol 17:38–56

Scott R, Thoner G (1986) Ego deficits in anorexia nervosa patients and incest victims: an MMPI comparative analysis. Psychol Rep 58:839–846

Selvini-Palazzoli M (1963) Self starvation. Human context books. Chaucer, London

Sherry D (1981) In: Cioffi LA, James WPT, Van Itallie TB (eds) The body weight regulatory system: normal and disturbed mechanism. Raven, New York

Stent GS (1978) Paradoxes of progress. Freeman, San Francisco, p 21

Tomkins SS (1962) Affect/imagery/consciousness, vol 1. The positive affects. Springer, Berlin Heidelberg New York

CHAPTER 10

Some Impressive Issues of Bizarre Character in the Life of Anorectics

We would like to describe some of the events in the daily life of various anorectics to further illustrate this condition for the researcher or clinician who does not have a great deal of specific experience with anorectics.

Typically, anorectics are 15–24-year-old women, characterized by extremely thin, emaciated bodies. Usually this thinness is not hidden by a special way of dressing; dark clothes are often worn. The skin of the extremities is rather cyanotic. Anorectics are especially characterized by their activity, which is not of an aimless nature. They sometimes hold a job.

If possible, anorectics try to stay in their parents' home. This is a very common characteristic of these young women who could (or should, one would think) live separately, but prefer to remain in their nuclear family. This may be because they fear living alone, though at the same time they fight desperately for independence and autonomy. It is as if they would like to stay in the womb and thus be protected from evil. This desire to remain at home may be understood as both sadistic and masochistic behavior. It is sadistic in the sense that the anorectic angers her parents by her eating rituals and behavior, with her compulsive weighing, calculating, and preparing, and by her subservient attitude. Parents do not understand this self-destructive and self-humiliating behavior. It frightens them and they feel completely incompetent and impotent to deal with the situation. Many anorectics menace their parents with implicit or explicit suicide threats. The parents are therefore kept in a state of constant tension and anxiety.

The masochistic aspect of staying at home is demonstrated in the Cinderella role that many anorectics take on. They experience pleasure in enacting a role of humility and subservience. Masochism is also expressed by the renouncement of any drive pleasure and any satisfaction. Social activity is curtailed, since by not satisfying the existing hunger it becomes impossible for object relations with friends to be satisfied. This masochism is also shown in the renunciation of sexual activity, and usually even of masturbatory activity.

Anorectics are known to be prone to moodiness and are easily angered, although not by their own appearance, which is denied. They can, however, be angered by remarks about their looks or their lack of femininity. Their moodiness may be expressed by autoaggression in temper tantrums, by throwing themselves on the floor, by banging their heads against the wall, and by suicide attempts.

Some anorectics with a more differentiated character structure of a hysteric or borderline nature may play a certain unfeminine or malicious role when challenged. This took place, for example, with two of my patients who, independently of one another (at different times and places), dressed like witches. One of the women was always dressed in black, including long black gloves and powdered her face a stark white, in order to produce a *femme fatale* effect. The other dressed similarly and in addition would emit strange screams. This similarity may be due to the fact that anorectics, though they discard their sex role and choose not to assume a male role, sometimes pattern themselves nonetheless on a symbol of female power – the witch.

I have already mentioned elsewhere that some anorectics eat an apple in bed seemingly with pleasure. Others chew gum incessantly. One girl I treated not only chewed about 60 daily, but also swallowed many of them intentionally, probably in order to express her rebellion and masochism. Some anorectics bite their nails, sometimes swallowing the bits. There are several possible explanations for the need of some anorectics to chew. There is certainly an aspect of aggressive pleasure in chewing, especially when one is fantasizing about chewing a certain object or person. This may be part of the general symbolic pattern of aggression. Biting nails and swallowing the bits also has an element of self-mutilation.

There may also be an element of exaggeration in this need to chew and an attempt to give an impression of vileness. I have seen this phenomenon quite often in drug-dependent persons, who may exaggerate to a great degree. It seems as if they must show how much more horrible they are than the average controlled person. The same applies to many anorectics who brag in a paradoxical way about their exaggerated behavior.

A final point may be that many anorectics, being hyperactive, feel a need to keep the mastication masculature active as well.

Some patients show other elements of infantile regression. For example, certain anorectics show a clear gastrocolic reflex. This is usually observed in infants, who when drinking milk immediately start to defecate. As the stomach is filled there is a reflex causing increased colon motiltiy and speedy evacuation. Though this reaction is also found in certain highly sensitive adults, anorectics seem to have a similar gastrocolic reflex because the gastrointestinal system is their main and global expressive ground. We tend to refer to the various oral elements in these and other dyscontrol patients, but we should not forget that it is the entire digestive system which is resomatized, which has come to life as almost the only reacting system, in both symbolic, abstract, and concrete ways, and as an affect equivalent (obvious anal elements). Some patients take measures to avoid not only swallowing or digesting, but also to empty their gastrointestinal system and thus symbolically to purify their whole system.

These characteristics and expressions can be best illustrated in a description of one of my patients, an anorectic girl of 19 years of age. She was a very moody, depressed, and angry person who lived at her parents' home, causing them constant fear and tension. When angered, she would often bang her head like an infant and throw herself on the floor in impotent rage. Her parents were afraid to leave her at home by herself because she seemed to be accident prone.

One day it was reported to me that she had either jumped or fallen off the balcony of their fourth-floor apartment. She did not injure herself seriously since the incident took place in the wintertime and she had fallen into a puddle of water, which had probably softened the impact. In any event, she was immediately hospitalized in a neurosurgical department, as she had sustained some minor injury to one of her lower cervical vertebrae. The injury and subsequent treatment required her to lie in a supine, hyperextended postion, head upward. The girl's immediate reaction to this was to become extremely angry with her parents for not providing her a mirror system which would have allowed her to read in this uncomfortable position. Her anger was almost limitless. This reaction amazed everyone, whatever the reasons had been for this intended or unconsciously intended suicide. It was a clear example of a shift in the value system of anorectics, as I have claimed above, which produces a total denial of important incidents, almost like a *belle indifference* phenomenon.

Another example was a patient who was not a classic anorectic but more a typical bulimic, who nonetheless exhibited similar attitudes to anorectics. She was referred to me by her family doctor who thought she was an addict. Indeed, at least twice a week she took 200–250 tablets of a laxative drug at a time. Whenever she had taken the tablets she would sit for long hours at night on the toilet and the next morning would feel relieved, happy, and reborn. We verified that the medicine itself did not contain any harmful or addictive material. Nevertheless, her excessive behavior was a cause for concern.

In this specific case, many elements of voyeurism and exhibitionism could be seen. This was especially true of her dreams and fantasies, in which she carried out the intimate act of sitting on the toilet in public. She also had some sexual experiences which she submitted to with sadomasochistic fantasies. She expressed wishes by symbolic actions. At times, she not only swallowed everything (before taking the laxatives), but also could not prevent herself from stealing small items, as if to incorporate them. Her body build was quite normal, but, like many really thin anorectics, she spoke about wishing to cut off her perceived wide hips with a knife. When asked to draw her mother, she drew a neuter child, completely undifferentiated. She was not hyperactive, studied, and worked, but her feelings of inferiority in every respect brought her often to the brink of breaking down. Nevertheless, some aspects of her personality disorder were more healthy than those of the average anorectic. Her transference behavior had less acting out and resistance elements, and she improved remarkably well after a long period of treatment.

It would be possible to give many examples of anorectic behavior, but the many books which describe anorectic case studies make further description here unnecessary. What I intended to do was to give some examples of what I describe and claim to be the specific characteristic of anorectics, i.e., the excessive nature of their behavior disturbance. This is expressed by their continuous hunger, wanting, and wishing, and finally by their extreme self-control in holding back. Their hunger wishes are often expressed in a manner which escapes their internal censor. Anorectics express hunger drives by "nonrelevant" behavior in these bizarre excesses, childish in character. For anorectics, the excessive is expressed in conspicuous thinness, while the obese express this by animal-like devouring. Drug addicts, by excessive and bizarre behavior, play in some crazy way the role of those who can help themselves, like physicians. It therefore seems obvious that all dyscontrol syndromes are expressed in the very same way – through excessive behavior.

CHAPTER 11

Treatment

"The soul is born old, but it grows young – that is the comedy of life. The body is born young and grows old, that is life's tragedy."

Oscar Wilde: A Woman of No Importance III, 1893

A mode of treatment for anorexia nervosa has been suggested by every possible school of thought. Because no certain etiology has been established for this disorder, doctors are confused about rationalities of treatment. As with the uncertainty surrounding the use of polypragmasy, treatment multiplicity reflects the confusion, frustration, and lack of security surrounding this issue. The treatments suggested are intended both for hospital and for ambulatory or office settings.

These treatment procedures for anorexia are similar, in reasoning, purpose, and results, to those for other dyscontrol syndromes, especially drug abuse. In both instances, hospital treatment is only a temporary and emergency procedure to be applied in times of urgency, with the real treatment to be carried out later on an outpatient basis and for a much longer duration.

Hospital emergency treatment for the anorectic can be a life-saving procedure, with force-feeding sometimes being necessary in order to sustain life. For drug abusers, hospital treatment can be indirectly life saving by inducing withdrawal from the dangerous drug habit. In both cases, however, only the physical aspect of the disease is treated in hospital. The second part of the treatment for anorectics is long-term out-patient psychotherapy. For the drug abuser, it is the continuation of a comprehensive treatment program in the community and intensive individual or group psychotherapy. In both cases, hospital measures only will not keep the patient out of trouble for long.

Hospital Treatment for Anorectic Patients

Hospital treatment is necessary under specific conditions, such as when weight loss is between 25% and 40%. This rule is interpreted differently by various researchers, depending on the acuteness of the symptoms. Hospitalization may also be indicated when the first diagnostic considerations are verified. This is for the simple reason that under hospital conditions it is easier to examine all the different organic, endocrine, and biochemical elements, and to rule out any significant malfunctioning of the body.

Hospital treatment as such should be initiated as an emergency measure and then only depending on the patient's readiness to accept treatment. Patients are not usually very agreeable to being admitted to a psychiatric ward. Therefore, it is certainly helpful for the patients to meet a few of the staff of the department before admittance in order to establish both a personal rapport and to have explained in simple terms the kinds of treatment to be undertaken and the probable length of stay.

In very rare cases, it may be necessary to hospitalize a patient involuntarily because of her refusal of treatment and the real danger to her life. I am not one who believes that psychotherapy cannot be started while starvation effects are still prevalent. These effects need not interfere, nor need rigid dieting have antitherapeutic effects, in contrast to Russell's opinion (1981). We believe that hospital treatment can serve in the initiation of psychotherapy, and thus support primary motivating factors.

Hospital procedure should, when possible, not be opposed to a general treatment policy. It is not that we want to support a rebellious infantile attitude, but we do recognize and make the patients conscious of their rebellion against dependency, while not supporting the dependency needs they fight against in their bitter struggle for control. Using authoritative measures will perhaps cause a weight gain, but of those statistics which show weight gain by behavioral conditioning none show any improvement in emotional maturity, or in post-hospital behavior. Although hospital admission includes emergency measures for achieving quick weight gain, one has to be aware that this is achieved with a further loss of independence, freedom, and autonomy.

The therapist must decide if the patient's life is in danger, and must also consider whether forced hospitalization will lead to a subliminal involvement in a battle for power. On the one hand, the patient will gain a few kilograms when faced with authority, in order to get out of the hospital trap; on the other hand, these measures rightly induce the patient's perception of the therapist as nonempathic and punitive. This in turn causes regression and may destroy any chances for improvement of the patient through continuous therapy. Having long-term aims in mind, I would try not to force fast physical gain by such conditioning behavior, unless it were absolutely vital. It has been shown that supportive nursing care, modified bed rest, and a high caloric diet, together with other ward treatments, all within the context of a present- and future-oriented therapeutic approach, will do at least as much. Moreover, this approach will produce a much more mutually honest and trusting attitude, and will also leave the patient with some control (Garfinkel and Garner 1982). Treatment involving initial prolonged bed rest with a modest target for weight gain is supported by Crisp (1970) and Fox and James (1976).

In order not to lose their strict control, anorectic patients, when urged to give up many of their habits, may try to deceive, hide and hoard, vomit, or exercise in an exaggerated manner. These are signs that they feel on the verge of incompetence to deal with authority and that they need to keep some mastery to themselves under the pressure of the institution.

A treatment, therefore, which involves a dialogue between equals, in which the therapist, though he has knowledge nevertheless has no wish to use power, will be the most useful for setting up a positive working alliance. As with any rational formation of a working team with a common aim, the relation itself should be defined and both short-term and long-term aimes stipulated. One of the initial points of agreement should be that the patient should try not to lose any more weight. At the same time, the therapists should promise not to use any superfluous authoritative measures without preparing the patient and having her agreement. In this way a gradual trusting relationship can be established.

There is one exception to this procedure: when the patient is stubbornly resistant to any kind of communication, continues to lose weight, and possibly shows suicidal or psychotic behavior. At this point the patient must be treated against her will, and her family informed at the same time about this necessary step. Tube feeding, or preferably parenteral hyperalimentation will be instituted. The patient should also be informed about the treatment and the reasons for its urgency. The hospital staff must be careful not to let the patient gain too much weight in too short a time. A gradual weight gain is preferred both for physiologic considerations and because the patient has to adapt to the change in body image. I would consider this as one of the first steps of psychotherapy.

Liebman et al. (1974a, b) have shown the importance of contact by the therapist with the family, and stress the value of family therapy in the treatment of anorexia. Temporary success was achieved within weeks when family settings were combined with operant conditioning.

Pharmacologic Treatment

Many groups of drugs have been proposed for the treatment of anorexia, mostly from the arsenal of psychopharmacological substances. These are suggested in part because of their physiological effects. However, drug treatment generally can be detrimental to a later psychotherapeutic approach, and therefore its rationale should be considered from case to case. Major tranquilizers (neuroleptics) such as chlorpromazine or other phenothiazine compounds, and butyrophenones have been used by many clinicians. As early as 1958 they were introduced in treatment for anorexia by Dally (1958), and have been used ever since. Dosage varies considerably, but is usually high (up to 2000 mg chlorpromazine/day for instance). The effect of these drugs is usually anxiolytic and sedative; they help the patients to tolerate bed rest, decrease their resistance to eating, and finally possibly assist in weight increase due to their effect on catecholamines.

I have my doubts about these rather general assumptions concerning the benefit of tranquilizers in the treatment of anorexia. Tranquilizers are used to reduce anxiety and/or psychotic cognition, but, in contrast to other psychologic disorders, we feel that there is generally no overt anxiety in anorectic patients, apart from their fear of loss of control. It is this very fear of loss of control that the use of tranquilizers heightens. I learned this from several patients when I also experimented with medium doses of phenothiazines. One patient in particular expressed it so well that her words are still imprinted on my memory. She observed that on chlorpromazine administration she felt sedated, which in turn made her frightened that her control over her body would relax and then she would be even less able to master any impulses (Edelstein and Noy 1967). It is the disinhibition that is feared, and as a consequence, the patient tenses up even more and tries to resist the influence of the drug, which is possible to a certain degree.

Therefore, I believe that the administration of these drugs is actually antitherapeutic in the sense that they work against the trends of the personality. I thus claimed (Edelstein 1975) that psychoactive drugs must be administered only under very specific conditions and only in accordance with the coping devices of the patient. If an anorectic is trying to inhibit and master impulses, it is of no avail to give a drug which is releasing inhibitions and control. In such a vulnerable state, the patient will not be able to relax. Of course, if one chooses to administer very high doses one can shock a patient into a state of nonresistance. This can be done, however, only within the context of authoritarian methods. This is especially true when hospitalization is forced, posing a major threat to independence and autonomy. By adding drugs to this situation a feeling of loss of control and vulnerability is produced which causes double stress to the patient. Such a feeling of defeat will make it that much harder for the patient to form a constructive alliance with a therapist. Basic trust will be practically nonexistent and any authority will be seen as having a negative value.

Other authors (Halmi et al. 1983) recommend anti-depressant medication, which is sometimes justified since it produces an initial lessening of anxiety. It is also thought to be of benefit in treating the depressive symptoms that anorexia patients are assumed to exhibit. Nevertheless, I argue that the elements which might be seen as depressive are in fact evidence of a character deviation toward masochistic, even ascetic trends.

Any artificial stimulation of appetitive or weight gain would only work against the patient's motivation to master bodily needs. This is often the case with the use of appetite-stimulating drugs such as cyproheptadine which, as with other drug treatments, only heighten the patient's own struggle to control physical impulses. It is not true that the anorectic does not feel hunger or has no appetite; instead the patient is fighting these impulses or impulse satisfactions. Therefore, we ought not to commit the simple mistake of using treatments and drugs to induce the feelings which the patient is trying to fight or control, especially if we hope to use more than simple first-aid measures. An interesting use of both antipsychotics and antidepressants in treatment of anorectics was described by Biebl (1986) as an initial and individual way of dealing with the patient's coping mechanisms by influencing her ergotropic and trophotropic systems.

Psychotherapy

Fundamentals

The controversy over the optimal kind of treatment for anorectics has yet to be settled. On a hospital ward, group therapy can be of value. Edelstein and Moguilner (1987) have shown that there is a rationale for homogeneous groups of anorectics. Anorectics often deny their own body forms, and this is often reinforced by positive delusional elements (as has also been found with cancer patients, see Edelstein et al. 1988). Confrontation with other anorectic patients can be of help in the formation of dialogue, through which the patients are able gradually to perceive their own body images in more realistic form.

There are certainly other elements which make group therapy amenable, such as the basic feeling of sharing similar experiences or modes of expression of emotional origin. This decreases the need for shame, humiliation, and isolation.

Treatment through family therapy has met with much enthusiasm and reported success. Minuchin et al. (1978) and Selvini-Palazzoli (1978), as mentioned above, have introduced this approach, seeing the anorectic's behavior as a family barometer. A particular family style, which encourages the anorectic to assume a special role, is seen as a specific factor. For example, an overprotective family may have discouraged the search for autonomy. Minuchin has remarked that: "[The anorectic's] overinvolvement with her family handicaps her involvement with the extrafamilial world, causing a developmental lag." In such a family situation there will be much unconscious ambivalence concerning the "wished-for" independence of the anorectic adolescent. In family therapy, the members of such "quiet" families can learn more about each other and their enmeshment and mutual intrusions. The patient's symptoms can be redefined and everybody encouraged to express emotions more openly.

Selvini-Palazzoli (1978) has suggested that a common characteristic in families with an anorectic member is the "disqualification" of communication. This means that a message is being sent on one level, while being rejected, denied, or qualified on a different level. She also points to the existence of "positive connotation," by which she attributes "constructive intentions to the kind of interpersonal behavior, that is commonly described as destructive and injurious."

It seems that this kind of comprehensive and open approach by an experienced therapist and a motivated family can open up a wide spectrum of direct communications and a general improvement in the patient.

Individual Psychotherapeutic Approaches

My own suggestion for therapy is based on my belief concerning the motivating circumstances that produce anorectic behavior. This must begin with a basic respect for the patient's abilities and modes of dealing with internal and external conflicts and crises. In other words, I try to understand the type of coping devices prevalent and to see why that particular "choice" of seemingly deviant devices had been made. The ego strength available to the patient must next be evaluated. This is to judge whether the patient will have the motivation and strength to gradually change attitudes and coping devices in order to live a more functional life, with better identity and object relations, and to be able to depersonalize food, which has itself been serving as an object.

As in all dynamic therapies one should deal first with the defenses, making the patient more conscious of them through confrontation or interpretation. Only at a later stage should the affects themselves be dealt with. The therapist must be aware that affects are very touchy and overwhelming subjects, otherwise those rigid defenses would not be so rigid. This is especially true with the denial of positive "good" affects and the conspicuousness of the "evil" affect, as with aggression turned upon the body, expressed as masochism and asceticism. There is also the more covert aggression and anger felt towards the mother and the family, as well as against female sexuality altogether. It is a lack of defusion between love and hatred toward the incorporated, devoured mother figure. In addition, there is the affectively ambivalent feeling toward the personalized object – food.

Altogether, a defense against any sign of affect, by the striving for absolute autonomy and independence, is apparent. The not-giving-in attitude itself is a defense against emotionality. Needs, both great and small, are felt all the time and are rejected. This is because needs stand somewhere between impulse and emotionality; they are constantly present and cause a striving for fulfillment. This is one of the unlimited desires of the body that the anorectic has to control, because need satisfaction may be not possible. For the anorectic, need is sex, which is corporal and shameful. If needs are not fulfilled one is independent of both bodily needs and impulses. This is seen by the anorectic as real control. The anorectic strives for omnipotent mastery of the weak body and its needs, and for its recreation as a strong body, able to withstand any test. So fulfillment is also symbolized or concretized by filling – the body – and this can be denied in the most concrete sense. Therefore, the anorectic is in complete control, since needs are no longer felt. By feeling no hunger the anorectic feels no satiety, thus rejecting the female role which is seen as a hunger for sex, satisfaction, satiety, and fulfillment. This dynamic can also be acted out in the therapeutic relationship towards the therapist. The anorectic is very strongly resistant to therapy to show her resistance against needs, in this case dependency needs. It is a curious fact that by her fragile bodily appearance the anorectic projects both an image of dependence on people, and an image of an independent, disciplined Spartan who can exist in such an emaciated state.

As well as deciding on the type and course of therapy to be followed, therapists must also be aware of their own feelings and associations, especially when dealing with anorectic patients. When seeing a potential patient for the first time, a therapist will usually be aware of the patient's face, features, gestures, and nonverbal behavior. However, when dealing with dyscontrol syndromes such as anorexia nervosa, obesity, and drug abuse there are certain features of the body and behavior which strike a therapist at the very first glance. These aspects of behavior and bodily appearance may arouse negative feelings or moral judgments in the therapist. I would not call this countertransference, as it is experienced by the therapist during the first minutes of seeing a patient, before any real discourse, dialogue, or therapeutic relationship has been established. It is more the result of an image we all have of normal body build, which encourages the idea of certain stereotypes of the human figure. For example, when we see someone with a very emaciated, skeleton-like body, who nonetheless exhibits not suffering but stubbornness, we may feel pity and also disgust, which are responses to the inability to grasp this enormous self-punishing behavior. The experience may arouse associations with the infamous appearance of concentration camp inmates, provoking us to anger and to say, "What right do they have to look like or imitate those poorest of suffering humans?" The self-inflicted quality of the disorder can anger us as well as we may feel that doctors have enough work fighting diseases of a "real" nature. We may also initially feel pity for the family which is permanently suffering pain and anxiety.

Our prior knowledge of this disease can cause us to think immediately of patients' stubbornness and lack of motivation, of the danger to life, possible empathy, and whether we will have the ability to really empathize with the potential patient. The therapist may then begin to think about the low success rate and lengthy treatment process, in which unbelievable tolerance and patience are needed. This may lead the therapist to question whether the patient is not in fact suffering from some physical element that the doctors could have missed, thereby harming the patient.

Among other considerations of the therapist's ability to treat anorectic patients would be whether the first messages of the delusional body image are received, and how they are dealt with. This response immediately raises doubts as to the therapist's ability to empathize with, identify with, or rationally understand the anorectic. The anorectic's forbidding asexual attitude may also cause the therapist to feel aggression, anger, and a readiness to fight, to meet omnipotence with omnipotence.

In a similar way, therapists will have to check their inherent reactions and feelings when dealing with other kinds of dyscontrol syndromes, especially obesity and drug abuse. I believe that the therapeutic community idea is used when saying that people suffering from dyscontrol syndromes are not good candidates for psychotherapy. This is usually said after estimating ego strength, motivation, and other factors. But I believe, that in these cases, as with anorectic patients, the therapist has first of all to overcame certain biases or attitudes before considering candidacy for treatment. As stated above, the therapist must then overcome certain personal elements which may affect his ability to treat these patients.

In an effort to clarify the possible situation when dealing with dyscontrol syndromes, I will next describe certain unconscious attitudes, feelings, and biases which the therapist may experience when confronted by the obese and drug abusers as candidates for therapy. As with the anorectic, the obese patient presents the analyst with an unusual situation where the patient expresses conflicts through self-induced symptoms instead of through psychic signs such as anxiety. Secondly, the immediacy of the patient's physical non-normally makes the situation unusual. Certain characteristics which are normally associated with the obese can influence a therapist's ability to see the patient in an objective light. These characteristics include the belief that overweight people are friendly and happy. We may see an element of sloppiness and an attitude of letting-go, and may find the perceived lack of self-discipline and inability to control impulses as infantile and meriting disgust. We may believe that they should be doing something more mature than eating. The therapist also often has difficulty with the "as-if obvious" nature of dyscontrol syndromes. When working with other categories of patients a sudden insight into infantile behavior or archaic defenses is usually arrived at only after hard mutual work. With the obese, however, the behavior and defense lie, so to speak, on the surface where they can be unmasked and observed from the beginning, showing how infantile and orally regressed this potential patient is. This, I believe, is one of the aspects therapists dislike most in dealing with patients with dyscontrol syndromes. This may also occur in conjunction with more personal memories and associations of the therapist concerning obese persons in their own families or social life. These thoughts and fantasies might take place before anything has been said between the therapist and the patient.

With the drug abuser, though the success rate of analytic or other psychodynamic therapy is not lower than for other dyscontrol syndromes, the literature describes these personalities as psychopathic or character disorders who should be avoided. Drug abusers arouse immediate associations of danger, murder, aggression, and desperation to do anything to get the drug. With these patients the initial effort is usually greater since they (and of course the therapist) must first be motivated. Value judgments may come to mind, such as believing that these are people who usually do not work, feel no responsibility, have little patience or tolerance, and may be immediately acting out. I imagine that therapists are also not completely free of vague fears concerning drugs and the feelings or states they induce (Edelstein 1975). Even the different and unique social status of the drug abuser may play a role in influencing a therapist's thoughts and feelings of rejection. In this case it is not so much the deviant body that disturbs the therapist, but more the knowledge that the body is being mysteriously influenced and driven by some drug and that the therapist is incompetent to deal with it. Only after confronting these preconceived notions can the therapist apply more rational considerations concerning ego strength, the amount of superego existing, whether empathy could be felt or developed, and, finally, prognostic factors.

The therapist must be conscious of all these initial biases when considering the treatment of patients suffering from anorexia, obesity, or drug addiction. Therapy is a very intense process, requiring endurance, tolerance, and the empathy to persevere with the patient through any and all regressions. Therefore the therapist must not only motivate the patient for a long treatment, but must also motivate himself. This entails accepting the patient for him- or herself, while recognizing the many unconscious resistances on the part of the therapist.

Therapists must also avoid splitting treatment between the body and the mind. This is especially necessary when dealing with patients who use their bodies to express psychologic disorders. The traditional line has been that food disorders, since they affect the body, should be treated only by physicians. The psychotherapist was supposed to deal only with the emotional aspect by psychotherapy. In cases of dyscontrol syndrome, however, the patient is actually using splitting as a main mechanism, and therefore we propose as far as possible not to divide the work between an internist and psychotherapist. The only exception envisaged would be where a nurse or dietician was involved in treatment.

In Chapter 9 we tried to show the splitting mechanism of the ego and the denial used by the anorectic. Splitting is a very important mechanism in the anorectic allowing defusion of body and soul, and the use of the body as a representational object. The real self can be split from the false self that is being played with and demonstrated. Drives, such as sex and hunger drives which are the most vital of all, are split off from consciousness, or at least isolated and denied. The anorectic is therefore living with her body as a kind of object, which is also seen as being a subjective body in the sense that it belongs to her and by which she devours those parental figures she ambivalently loves and hates, fuses with and destroys.

One of the aims of therapy should be to abolish this split so that the patient will learn not to alienate her body or hide behind her "false" self, in order to discover that there are real objects which one does not have to be threatened by.

The anorectic needs to learn to relate to an integrated body-mind self. Therefore, the therapist must be able to demonstrate to the patient that he relates to more than just a split-off part of the patient, and, further, that he relates out of respect and a sense of empathic understanding. It is for this reason that I am against splitting treatment between internist and psychotherapist. Also Thomä (1977), although he recommends combined treatments, points out the difficulties split treatment can produce in intrastaff relations.

Therefore, the therapist cannot serve as a model for a double bind message. The therapist must treat the whole person and be a whole person in his approach to the patient. He should show a tolerant acceptance of the difficulties with a clear expression of time limitation, which will encourage the patient to see therapy as a process of development and growth with various phases and aspects. This acceptance of the present situation must be honestly felt, though it does not preclude changes in attitudes on both sides. Nevertheless, the therapist should also make it clear that he will not be integrated or incorporated into the patient's world. This is especially necessary with anorectic patients, since the "hunger ideology" includes both the wish to devour and the resistance to that wish.

Stated in very general terms, one of the attainments of such an attitude which is tolerant but depends on development is the expectation that the patient will be able to move from somatization to desomatization. This means that the patient will be able to relearn to express feelings instead of manipulating body parts or just stating sensations. The patient must learn to believe that this ability to express feelings can be achieved without becoming dependent and losing autonomy. As with any psychosomatic patient, one should strive for the psychic expression of emotions and affect in general.

The other aspect of treatment is the supporting of verbalization, in contrast to the deverbalization which had taken place. Body language, which is used to express isolation, will be gradually abolished. Later, body language should be ego syntonic and integrated into a more unified organismic whole. Another major aim is the clarification of the defenses used against female identity. Identity formation is certainly disturbed in these patients and this disturbance is reinforced by social, cultural, and possibly even religious factors. This is shown by punitive, masochistic, and often ascetic attitudes in adolescence. Adolescence, a period of extreme changes in self-assertion and of moving into adult society, is characterized by a constant battle between erotic impulses and counterattitudes of discipline, self-discipline, and castigation. Feelings of happiness, the wish to let go, and the need for self-control are typical of that period.

For the anorectic, the fulfillment of these needs produces the fear of dependency, which the anorectic deals with by expressing no needs at all. The state of having no needs, of sacrifice, masochism, and even asceticism creates a sense of autonomy, as well as mastery and omnipotence. The characteristics of hypervitality and hyperactivity may be understood as symptoms of the striving to overcome the feeling of deadness and emptiness inside, again by overcontrol and reversal.

This control takes the place of fulfilling, or filling the body, which symbolically and concretely would risk becoming dependent; continued stimulation would end in satisfaction, with drive wishes gratified which she, in her fantasy, will not be able to inhibit or eventually prevent.

This thought leads us to the concept of inner space, which in the anorectic is greatly feared. The anorectic neither wants nor dares to fill that inner space, lest it should cause inevitable growth. The sensed emptiness also gives the anorectic an experience of sensuous pleasure.

Usually after a long period of therapy in which the anorectic learns to perceive her body differently, female identity becomes less feared and will be accepted to a greater degree. With this acceptance the deviations of delusional quality toward the body as an outside object will lessen also. It is as if the fantasized danger had gone, and with it, all defences against it disappear as well. Usually the last issue able to be changed in any degree is the attitude to real object relation. It is in this final stage that the body and food are relinquished as objects or transitional objects.

Of course, this process may take a very long time, years in fact, years with regressions and progress, with acting out and failures. Anger and aggression will be common and there may be impotent rage on both sides. One very important point is that the therapist must be able to show the patient how not to be afraid of impulses while at the same time leaving the patient with the feeling that her control is not completely superfluous and is of a permanent nature.

No doubt other treatment methods are applicable, such as cognitive-behavioral methods or suggestive devices. However, different methods should not be used by different therapists on one patient at the same time. Garfinkel and Garner (1982) describe at least 30 various papers dealing with operant conditioning, reinforcements, behavior therapy – in general, the methods of reward and punishment.

Therapeutic Results: Outcome

Bemporad and Ratey (1985) have demonstrated certain parental patterns, especially of fathers toward their daughters who later became anorectic. In particularly, they treated so-called postanorectic girls and found similar characteristics in them all, although their fasting behavior had ceased. In our own experience with about 12 such postanorectic women, we still found signs of regressive characteristics, but some more healthy object relations. Their eating patterns improved and their attitude towards spiritual values was still very high. As a result of therapy it seems that postanorectic women show a marked improvement in their attitude to female identity and erotic feelings. Nevertheless, it is our impression that in spite of almost complete improvement, their attitude to their body image remained distorted. These women still saw themselves as having normal or overweight body types.

Another interesting, important improvement or change is the disappearance of their previous hyperactivity. This may be a sign that the necessity to prove themselves omnipotent has decreased.

I propose the use of more intensive, instead of extensive, process descriptions, which might teach us more about the dynamics of the disease.

Supporting these findings is a study by Hall and Crisp (1987) who compared the outcome of "dietary advice patients" and those under psychotherapy. The dietary advice group showed significant weight gain, whereas the dynamically oriented psychotherapy group (individual and family) made significant improvement in sexual and social adjustment. Other follow-up studies with good detailed evaluations have been collected and reviewed by several authors. For example, Hsu (1980) selected 16 studies, leaving out many others from his review since he found they contained serious failings. He listed the possible results of therapy as various symptoms:

1. Mortality
2. Nutritional outcome
3. Menstrual outcome
4. Eating difficulties at follow-up
5. Psychiatric outcome
6. Psychosexual outcome
7. Psychosocial outcome
8. Effects of treatment (cannot be gauged)

Hsu was not able to arrive at a meaningful evaluation of the results of this review in the various fields of behavior.

In his own study, Hsu (1980) claimed that approximately 40% of the anorectics he studied recovered spontaneously from an eating disorder episode during adolescence. A further 20% responded to treatment, leaving 40% of cases with chronic anorexia, with varying course development.

Another follow-up study of Steinhausen and Glanville (1983) reviewed 45 studies from the years 1953–1981. They focused in particular on two themes: the effectiveness of different methods of treatment and the identification of prognostic factors. Steinhausen also detailed and differentiated the various elements as in Hsu's study. It seems very difficult to estimate the rate of improvement, as definitions vary enormously – the published rates of improvement vary between 10%–86%, the majority being between 30%–50%.

One of the greatest difficulties is that the division into various factors demonstrates certain aspects of behavior, which may or may not become normalized under certain focused modes of treatment. These elements can be used as favorable or unfavorable prognostic factors. However, it will certainly be necessary in the future to relate to general psychopathology, personal dynamics, and personality (dealing with internal and external aspects, as well as with psychosocial elements and adjustment). Then follow-up studies can be undertaken in a unidimensional way.

Studies which deal with outcome try to compare concrete elements which can be easily measured and reported, such as weight and menstruation. Morgan and Russell (1975) conducted such a study and could thus introduce categories such as "good," "intermediate," and "poor." However, as shown before, there are other elements which should be measured in order to arrive at concrete conclusions concerning the whole syndrome.

Two statistical studies (Hiroyuki et al. 1985; Suematsu et al. 1985) concerning the occurrence and prognosis of anorexia in Japan demonstrate the interest and attention this disorder has created there lately, where its occurrence seems to be causing concern to the public and to clinical institutions.

Reviewing and analyzing follow-up studies is very important. In this way we can examine the natural history of the disease, its duration, and the influence of treatment on duration. We can also learn from such studies which modes of therapy will influence which elements and symptoms of this complex disease. However, we also have to be aware that there is as yet no unified view of anorexia so that different researchers will lay different stress on different elements. We shall have to learn to differentiate between signs and symptoms, and their meaning in connection with the regression or the coping ability of the patient. In other words, we shall have to estimate not only concrete behavioral or physical symptoms, but also evaluate adaptive and maladaptive measures in the process of therapeutic experience.

References

Bemporad JR, Ratey J (1985) Intensive psychotherapy of former anorexic individuals. Am J Psychother 39(4):454–466

Biebl W (1986) Anorexia nervosa. Enke, Stuttgart, pp 210–211

Crisp AH (1965) Clinical and therapeutic aspects of anorexia nervosa: a study of thirty cases. J Psychosom Res 9:67–78

Crisp AH (1970) Premorbid factors in adult disorders of weight, with particular reference to primary anorexia nervosa (weight phobia): a literature review. J Psychosom Res 14:1–22

Dally PJ, Oppenheim GB, Sargant W (1958) Anorexia nervosa. Br Med J 2:633–634

Edelstein EL (1975) Elaborations on the meaning of repetitive behavior in drug dependent personalities. Br J Addict 70:365–373

Edelstein EL, Moguilner E (1986) Homogeneous group therapy in anorectic patients. Psychother Psychosom 8:205–208

Edelstein EL, Noy P (1967) Psychiatric drug treatment: personality factors and dynamic aspects. Psychosomatics 8:222–226

Edelstein EL, Nathanson DL, Stone A (1988) Denial: theoretical aspects and research. Plenum, New York

Fox KC, James NM (1976) Anorexia nervosa: a study of 44 strictly defined cases. N Z Med J 84:309–312
Garfinkel PE, Garner DM (1982) Anorexia nervosa: a multidimensional perspective. Brunner/Marzel, New York
Hall A, Crisp AH (1987) Brief psychotherapy in the treatment of anorexia nervosa: preliminary findings in England. Br J Psychiatry 151:185–191
Halmi KA, Eckert E, Falk JR (1983) Cyproheptadine, an antidepressant and weight-inducing drug for anroexia nervosa. Psychopharmacol Bull 19:103–105
Hiroyuki S, Kuboki T, Itoh T (1985) Statistical studies on the prognosis of anorexia nervosa. Psychother Psychosom 43:104–112
Hsu LKG (1980) Outcome of anorexia nervosa. A review of the literature (1954–1978). Arch Gen Psychiatry 37:1041–1046
Liebman R, Minuchin S, Baker L (1974a) An integrated treatment program for anorexia nervosa. Am J Psychiatry 131:432–436
Liebman R, Minuchin S, Baker L (1974b) The role of the family in the treatment of anroexia nervosa. J Am Acad Child Psychiatry 13:264–274
Minuchin S, Rosman BL, Baker L (1978) Psychosomatic families: anorexia nervosa in context. Harvard University Press, Cambridge, p 60
Morgan HC, Russell GFM (1975) Value of family background and clinical features as predictors of long-term outcome in anorexia nervosa: four year follow-up study of 41 patients. Psychol Med 5(4):355–371
Russel GFM (1981) The current treatment of anorexia nervosa. Br J Psychiatry 138:164–166
Selvini-Palazzoli M (1978) Self-starvation – from individual to family therapy in the treatment of anorexia nervosa, 2nd edn. Aronson, New York
Steinhausen HC, Glanville K (1983) Editorial: follow-up studies of anorexia nervosa. A review of research findings. Psychol Med 13:239–249
Suematsu H, Ishikawa H, Kuboki T, Itoh T (1985) Statistical studies on anorexia nervosa in Japan: detailed clinical data on 1,011 patients. Psychother Psychosom 43:96–103
Thomä H (1973) Die Psychoanalyse der anorexia nervosa. Internist (Berlin) 13:437–442
Thomä H (1977) On the psychotherapy of patients with anorexia nervosa. Bull Menninger Clin 41(5):437–452

Epilogue

Integration and differentiation in an organism are opposed faces of a unitary growth process, even when growth is not in linear progression. Our conceptualization of anorexia nervosa touches on both these aspects and seems to be organically justified. Anorexia nervosa is a hunger disease that is well differentiated within the spectrum of dyscontrol syndromes. However, it is also a good example of a severe psychological maturation defect and its compensating control mechanisms, all well integrated within a somatic core with the tendency to achieve homeostasis and good coping.

In the formative years of adolescence one is aware of continuous oscillations and changes within the context of biological maturation. Growth and differentiation indicate progression but do not preclude regression. In this period of life, a pleasurable experience may cause fear of the hedonic experience itself, its repetition and its uncontrollable peaks. Hunger, in all its implications, represents desired and forbidden lust. It is preferable to feel satiated before hunger has arisen.

Consequently, one can observe the achievement of some mastery even over the autonomous system, including the pituitary-hypothalamic axis. This mastery is expressed in functional units. In some seemingly parallel way, psychological coping with the internal forces and external reality expresses itself in behavior which is apparently deviant but indicative of the direction of sublimatory possibilities. The mastery seems to be a continuous battle between drive strength and ego control. Control relates explicitly to hunger and implicitly to any desire, particularly to sexual drive. Control, then, is needed for any vital issue. In the various dyscontrol states control can be lax, extremely severe, or expressed in various sorts of deviant, rebellious behavior. All of these expressions also have interpersonal and intrafamilial connotations. These deviant inhibitions may contribute to the creation of a masochistic character structure and to severe regression from adult object relations.

We have tried to demonstrate the interconnections between anorexia nervosa, obesity, and drug abuse. The connections are in the inner core of ill-control on autonomous mechanisms and the expression of this ill-control in certain behavior. These three disorders are similar in that for the physician they are not real diseases, since they are self-produced. Regarding treatment motivation and treatment success they also present close similarities.

There is a very close connection between psychological coping and physiologic mechanisms as well as deviant social behavior. These close interconnections in all three illnesses present us with problems in the conceptualization of symbolism and meanings as well as in new and efficient therapeutic approaches.

Subject Index

GPSR Compliance

The European Union's (EU) General Product Safety Regulation (GPSR) is a set of rules that requires consumer products to be safe and our obligations to ensure this.

If you have any concerns about our products, you can contact us on ProductSafety@springernature.com

In case Publisher is established outside the EU, the EU authorized representative is:

Springer Nature Customer Service Center GmbH
Europaplatz 3
69115 Heidelberg, Germany

Batch number: 10844827

Printed by Printforce, the Netherlands